Contents

The Nature and Temperament of Foods ... 2

Overview of Temperaments ... 7

Melancholic ... 8

Sanguine ... 13

Choleric ... 18

Phlegmatic ... 22

Guidelines for Eating ... 49

Four Temperaments Test ... 51

Herbal Tea ... 54

The Nature and Temperament of Foods

The Connection between Human Nature, Temperament and Food.

Polymath Avicenna (980–1037 AD) expanded the theory of temperaments to encompass "emotional aspects, mental capacity, moral attitudes, self-awareness, movements and dreams". Temperaments are biologically based and help us understand personalities because they are believed to be directly linked to the human personality.

Avicenna believed that certain human moods, emotions and behaviors were caused by an excess or lack of bodily fluids called humors. Types of humors are blood, yellow bile, black bile, and phlegm. Every human has a different composition of these four types of humors. This is important because all aspects of our lives are influenced by the makeup of our bodies. The type of food we eat can have a significant impact on all of our organs and nerves from the brain to the heart, stomach, liver, kidneys and colon. Eating a poor diet can have enormous consequences. In the simplest cases, one can observe for example, the consumption of sugar that immediately produces acne. This is the body's response to the food consumed.

Poor nutrition can have affect our bodies very negatively. When we perpetually eat high levels of the wrong foods or do not get enough of the nutrients we need, this can cause changes to sleep patterns, create nervousness, memory impairment, impaired digestion, excretion disorders, and skin complications, in addition to showing adverse effects on the liver, heart and reproductive organs. Many other things affect our overall health, including what we drink, our clothing materials, the air quality, amount of rest, and bowel movements.

Our neurological and psychiatric health are also directly affected by these external and internal factors. Since all of these factors are connected, it is imperative to understand the optimal nutrition necessary to create a normal, healthy life and weight, as well as peace of mind. This is possible when we understand our unique temperament or nature.

Every person has a unique humoral constitution which represents his healthy state. In order to maintain or achieve the correct humoral balance there is a power of self-preservation or adjustment called vital force in the body. If this power weakens, imbalance in the humoral composition is bound to occur and this causes disease. When this makeup is understood and the proper foods are consumed, it will help the body to regain this power and it will bring it to an optimum level and thereby restore humoral balance and good health. Also, a proper diet and good digestion will help maintain humoral balance.

The concept of humoral balance originated from the ancient Iranian civilization and was established upon the basic concept of temperament. Essentially temperament is developed as a result of the interaction of different elements in the human body. The interaction of these elements also affects the normal physical and emotional characteristics as well as the physiological functions of the body.

What we discover is that each person has a unique characteristic called temperament which is recognized and classified by his or her morphological, physiological and psychological features. A person is considered to be in a healthy state when his or her temperament maintains balance and most of the diseases occur when temperament becomes imbalanced. It is believed that no one temperament is exactly like any other, each is completely unique.

There are four general temperaments that characterize each individual that we will discuss in detail. They are Sanguine, Choleric, Melancholic and Phlegmatic. Each one of these temperaments may be defined by 4 conditions or a combination of them: warm, cold, moist and dry. When combined they are warm and moist; warm and dry: cold and moist; and cold and dry. In the context of this theory, each temperament/humor constitution is prone to specific diseases related to that temperament and some people may even require different treatments for the same disease depending on their temperament. Disease prevention and health care can be customized to each individual's temperament and will vary person to person.

Identifying a person's temperament is simple. A person's body temperature will help to identify temperament. Is your body typically hot or cold? One way to determine this is to evaluate how you dress in different seasons and temperatures. For example, in most weather conditions are you wearing excessive clothing, especially in summer? Those who have a cold disposition, do not tolerate the cold, and those who have a hot disposition do not tolerate the heat. In accordance with this principle 3 categories of people can be detected. The first are people who have cold temperament (cold-natured). They will generally be cold all the time and tend to wear more than clothing than others. The second are people with a hot temperament (hot-natured). And third are people who wear too much clothing in the winter and too little clothing in the summer.

Let's look at how our body temperature relates to the composition of the four humors in our bodies. According to Razi if you were to take a blood sample and to pour it into a glass container and leave it alone, after a time you can distinguish four layers.

A- The first layer (will be at the bottom, the darkest part). The bottom red layer contains the red blood cells (RBCs). If this is the predominant layer it will represent a SANGUINE temperament (characterized by hot & moist).
B- The second layer, the middle white layer, is composed of white blood cells (WBCs). If this is the predominant layer, this will

represent a PHLEGMATIC temperament (characterized by hot & dry).

C- The third layer is platelets. If this is the predominant layer, this will represent a MELANCHOLIC temperament (characterized by cold & dry).

D- The top layer is called plasma and forms about 60% of blood. If this is the predominant layer, this will represent a PHLEGMATIC temperament (characterized by cold & moist).

OVERVIEW OF TEMPERAMENTS

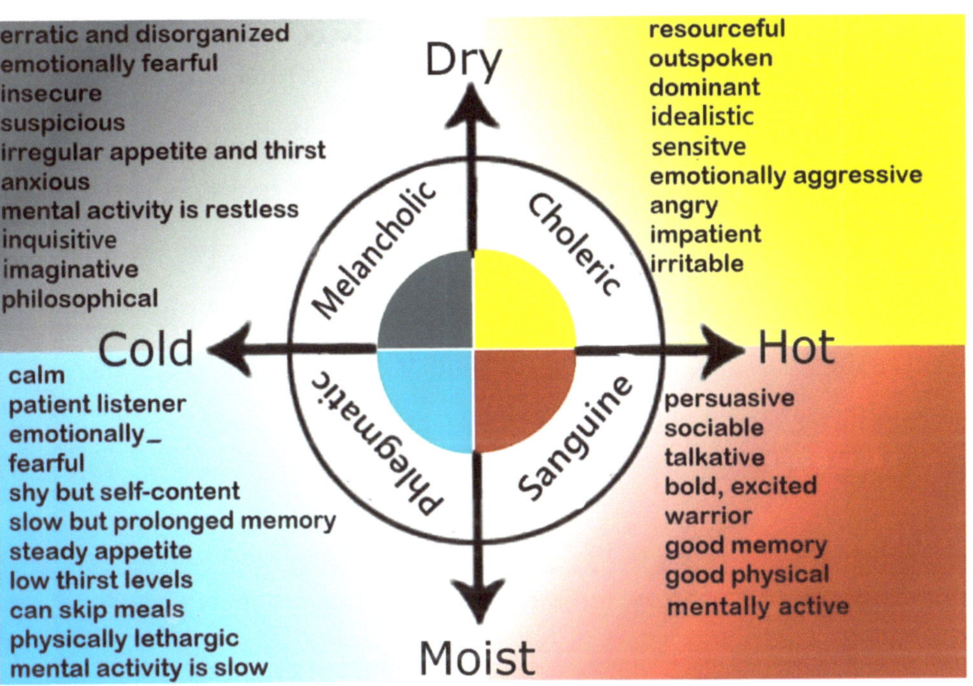

MELANCHOLIC

Introduction and General Considerations

Melancholia is a specific form of mental illness characterized by depressed mood, abnormal motor functions, and abnormal vegetative signs. A person whose constitution tended to have a preponderance of black bile had a melancholic disposition. In the complex elaboration of humorist theory, it was associated with "Earth" from the Four Elements of the Universe, the season of Autumn, the spleen as the originating organ and cold and dry as related qualities. In astrology it showed the influence of Saturn, hence the related adjective saturnine.

Being Cold and Dry in nature, the Melancholic Temperament is generally considered to be the most problematic of all the Four Temperaments, and the one most prone to pathology and disease. As the metabolic agent of the Earth element, Black Bile has a thickening, condensing effect on metabolic processes, and a Retentive virtue. Black Bile is also intimately involved in the formation of the hard, dense, solid structures and tissues of the body, such as bones, cartilage and connective tissue, as well as the nerves; all these parts of the body are Cold and Dry in nature, like Black Bile, and are prominent in those of a

Melancholic Temperament.

The delicate, colicky Melancholic digestion and Pepsis are notoriously difficult to treat and manage, and Melancholic individuals tend to have more food sensitivities, and are less tolerant of dietary abuses than any of the other Four Temperaments. Because Black Bile, the dominant humor in those of a Melancholic Temperament, receives the poorest and coarsest share of nutrients from food and drink, and is contrary in its basic qualities to the flourishing, nourishing Sanguine humor, Melancholic individuals need to take care to eat an adequately nourishing diet, having a sufficient amount of rich, unctuous, nutritious foods within a diet that is basically sound and balanced, and above all, their blood needs to be adequately nourished.

Melancholy people often experience the craving for sweets and starches as comfort foods, or to give them quick bursts of energy - this should be avoided, since it is no substitute for sound nutrition. They need to take care of their digestion and intestinal function on a daily basis, first and foremost through the food they eat. They need to get a good amount of fiber and bulk in their diet, and need to cook with a generous amount of aromatic, carminative herbs and spices, like Basil, Cumin, Dill, Sage, Fennel, Coriander, etc... A tea made from equal parts of Cumin, Coriander and Fennel seeds is a very soothing after dinner drink to help them relax.

Because the Melancholic Temperament is Dry in nature, drinking an adequate amount of water and fluids is a must. Exercise is a good way for Melancholic individuals to reduce their level of nervous stress and tension. Because they are prone to stiffness and tension in their muscles and tendons, bones and joints, stretching before a workout, to warm up, and especially after a workout, to cool down, are essential for them. Taking the time to engage in relaxation and deep breathing exercises before sleep is also great, as are foot massages with aromatic medicated balms and oils, to encourage deep, sound sleep. One of the best therapies for this is Oleation and Massage, which is called Abhyanga in Ayurvedic Medicine. Rolfing, or Deep Tissue Massage, also known as structural reintegration, is another great form of massage for those of a nervous or Melancholic Temperament.

Personal characteristics of the MELANCHOLY

They are deep and thoughtful, analytical, serious and purposeful, genius-prone, talented and creative, artistic or musical, appreciative of beauty, sensitive to others, self-sacrificing, conscientious, idealistic; as a parent, set high standards and want everything done right; as a homemaker, keep everything in order; as an employee, schedule-oriented and hard-working, a list maker and keeper, easily offended, can get too caught up in details, do not do well with change, struggle with insecurity, tend toward depression, but most organized people.

FOODS	Compatible	Inconsistent
VEGGIE	pumpkin, turnips, carrot, parsnips, kohlrabi, beetroot, asparagus	Potatoes, tomatoes, green beans, cucumber, eggplant, lemongrass, cilantro, cabbage, cauliflower, zucchini, mushrooms, green peas, sorrel, lettuce, okra, fava (broad beans), peas, butternut squash, wakame, endive
FRUITS	Avocado, grape, olive, banana, pineapple, papaya, mango, cantaloupe, lychee, jack fruit, mulberry, quince, Melon, cantaloupe, pear, avocado, cherries, pears, currants, raisins, grapes, white mulberry, cherry, berry, figs persimmons, melon gooseberry,	Lemon, lime, kiwi, plum, yellow plum, cherry, sour cherries, apricot, kumquat, watermelon, persics peach, medlar, sour pomegranate, orange, tangerine, grapefruit, barberry, strawberry, cranberry, sour plum, raspberry, stamps Hindi, buckthorn, hawthorn, dogwood, barberry, oak, all fruit sour, unripe fruit, silver berry, ziziphus, cornus mas, jujube, pitaya
HERBS		Coriander, spinach, purslane, opium poppy
GRAINS	Beans, pinto beans, red beans, black eye beans, red lentil, split pea, soy beans	Corn, millet, barley, lentils, beluga, mung beans, rice, hemp, rice, oats,
NUTS	Almonds, peanuts, sesame, sunflower seed	Chia, flixweed seeds, chestnut, hemp, pumpkin seeds
DAIRY		Cheese, old cheese, yogurt, milk
OILS	sesame oil, olive oil	
DRINKS	Grape juice, liqueur	Sour juices, teas especially strong tea, coffee, wines, ice, pickles, tomato sauce
SPICES		Stamp hindi, paste, lemon juice, verjuice, vinegar, dried limes, coriander, sumac, starch, white sugar
OTHER	Honey	

Melancholic diseases/conditions

Body fatigue, hemorrhoids, weight loss, depression, constipation dysuria gutierrez, sensation of burning when urinating, dark urine, vomit, black and tarry stools, leprosy, bad breath, dark eyes, dark-like night blindness, heartburn, overactive thoughts, sleep disruptions, loss of pleasure in all or most daily activities, nostalgia and restless. The appearance of black spots on the body, leprosy, skin diseases (soda), ulceration of the skin due to excessive itching, colic, colitis, forgetfulness and anemia or dementia, excessive greed, self-willed, fastidious habit; wistfulness, feeling anxious or irritable, appetites that go unsatisfied.

The list of conditions that the Melancholic Temperaments are potentially prone to is quite long: a delicate, colicky digestion with pronounced gas, distension, bloating, constipation and irritable bowel; nutrition and assimilation disorders and anemic conditions; nervous and neuromuscular conditions, and neurasthenia; arthritis and rheumatism; tremors, tics and spasms, insomnia and sleep disorders.

SANGUINE

Introduction and General Considerations

Blood, or the Sanguine humor, is Warm and Moist in temperament. It is Warm because it contains the Innate Heat of metabolism, as well as the Vital Force and other vital principles to power cellular metabolism. It is Moist because it is flourishing and nourishing, containing a rich supply of nutrients. A person whose constitution tended to have a preponderance of blood had a sanguine disposition. In the complex elaboration of humorist theory, it was associated with "Air" from the Four Elements of the Universe, the season of Spring, the spleen as the originating organ, and hot and moist as related qualities. In astrology it showed the influence of Jupiter.

Personal characteristics of the SANGUINE

They are tall and muscular and not thin. They have a full and strong heart rate, sleep well, and do not suffer from insomnia. Their skin is warm, moist and soft, and it is easier for them to tolerate the cold.

They crave sweet and sour foods, are fast and full of energy, passionate and have good libidos. They are susceptible to cardiovascular disease and high blood pressure. They are very intelligent with excellent memories.

They have a high-risk tolerance, are very creative, and are prone to pleasure-seeking behaviors. Their constant cravings may lead to overeating and weight problems, and they are likely to struggle with addictions. Their natural abilities will also serve them well if they choose jobs related to marketing, travel, fashion, cooking, sports, and the arts. Other characteristics include charming, cheerful, love people, energetic, talkative, passionate and compassionate, positive, sometimes unpredictable, expressive influencer, an excellent comedian, salesman or clown, quirky or eccentric and just plain fun.

Psychological Understanding and Management of the Sanguine Temperament:

Due to the moistness of the Sanguine nature, those of a Sanguine temperament are outgoing, social, ingratiating and gregarious. Due to the warmth of the Sanguine nature, they are also enthusiastic, curious expressive and joyful. In general, those of a Sanguine temperament tend to be hedonists and pleasure seekers, and have a low tolerance for asceticism, or for anything that is forced, unnatural or unpleasant. As such, any therapeutic measures or suggestions proposed for those of a Sanguine temperament must be made as pleasant and appealing as possible. Bitter medicines should be avoided, or made to taste more pleasant if at all possible. If exercise can be made into a social affair or a team sport, or into an aesthetically pleasing art form, such as dance, that will appeal to the Sanguine.

Instead of loneliness, drudgery and sacrifice, if what is good for you can also be made enjoyable and fun, this is the Sanguine preference. Sanguine types are not prone to excessive discipline or self- sacrifice, and will not force it on anyone else. Where some renunciation, discipline or self-sacrifice is required, the therapist must emphasize the greater payoffs or dividends to be reaped later on, and all the enjoyment and enrichment of life they will bring.

FOODS	Compatible	Inconsistent
VEGGIE	Potatoes, tomatoes, green beans, cucumber, eggplant, lemongrass, cilantro, cabbage, cauliflower, zucchini, mushrooms, green peas, sorrel, lettuce, okra, fava beans, peas, spinach, wakame, endive	Pumpkin, turnips, clover, cantaloupe, onions, garlic, horseradish, radishes, kohlrabi, beetroot, carrots, parsnips, turnips, olives, quince, asparagus
FRUITS	Lemon, lime, kiwi, plum, yellow plum, cherry, sour cherries, apricot, kumquat, watermelon, persics peach, medlar, sour pomegranate, orange, tangerine, grapefruit, barberry, strawberry, cranberry, sour plum, raspberry, stamps Hindi, buckthorn, hawthorn, dogwood, barberry, oak, all fruit sour, unripe fruit	Melon, cantaloupe, pineapple, pear, avocado, cherries, pears, banana, currants, olive, mango, grapes, white mulberry, mulberry, persimmons, gooseberry, dried apricot, papaya, jack fruit, quince
HERBS	Purslane, opium poppy	
GRAINS	Chia, flixweed seeds, chestnut, hemp, pumpkin seeds	Beans, pinto beans, red beans, black eye beans, red lentil, split pea, soy beans
NUTS	Almonds, peanuts, sesame, sunflower seed	Peanut, sunflower seeds, almonds, sesame
DAIRY	Whey	Butter, yogurt, fresh local cow's milk, sheep's milk
OILS	sesame oil, olive oil	
DRINKS	Sour juices, teas especially strong tea, coffee, wines, ice, pickles, tomato sauce	Grape juice, liquer
SPICES	Stamp hindi, paste, lemon juice, verjuice, vinegar, dried limes, coriander, sumac, starch	Black pepper, white pepper, cloves, ginger, fennel, mint, thyme, fennel, parsnip
OTHER		Honey, sugar, salt, condensed milk

Sanguine diseases/conditions

Heaviness of the head, yawning, sleeping, Kennedy's senses, sweet mouth, saliva (the viscous red color of the body), red tongue, tingling, boils and pimples on the body (especially on the forehead and back of the head and shoulders), gum and teeth bleeding, compulsive eating and excessive consumption of fried and spicy foods, circulation problems common, high blood pressure and migraine headaches. They are at risk for high fevers, cardiovascular problems such as arrhythmia, stroke or heart attack and even brain hemorrhages. Excess of yellow bile was thought to produce aggression, and excess anger reciprocally gave rise to liver derangement and imbalances in the humors.

CHOLERIC

Introduction and General Considerations

A person whose constitution tended to have a preponderance of yellow bile had a choleric associated disposition. In the complex elaboration of humorist theory, it was with "Fire" from the Four Elements of the Universe, the season of Summer, the spleen as the originating organ and hot and dry as related qualities. In astrology it showed the influence of Mars and the Sun. The Choleric Temperament has the nature of its associated element, Fire, and is Hot and Dry in its basic qualities. The dominant humor of the Choleric Temperament is the Choleric or Bilious humor, or Yellow Bile. Those of a Choleric temperament are fiery, high-energy people with a high level of Fire and Metabolic Heat in their bodies. They tend to be active, dynamic and athletic, having lean, wiry, muscular physiques, driving themselves hard to get the most that they can out of life, and quickly grow impatient. Their Hot, Dry natures make their skin warm, rough and dry to the touch, and makes muscles, veins and tendons well-defined. Choleric individuals tend to be intense, with a fiery sparkle in their eyes. They are dynamic, high- powered people, pushing to the limit to cram as much excitement and intensity into their life as they can. They have tons of energy and inspiration, they are pioneers, free-wheelers, the idea people, the brilliant, insightful creative movers and shakers who glow in the dark. Yellow Bile, their dominant humor, being hot, caustic, stimulating and provocative in nature, makes them bold, ambitious and audacious, courageous and proactive as their basic default state of spirit and being. They are rigorous and demanding.

The Choleric temperament is Hot and Dry, so their best diet is eating lots of Cold, Wet foods. They also need to stay well- hydrated and drink a lot of water and fluids.

This benefits them because of their powerful digestive juices, and because fresh fruits and vegetables have such a beneficial cooling, moistening and alkalizing/detoxifying effect on their bodies.

Anger and stress management, and learning how to control one's temper, can be another problem area on which Choleric individuals need to focus. Meditation and yoga are helpful calming and stress-relieving activities to engage in that have helped many Choleric individuals cool down and find peace within. Ideal jobs for them are: management, technology, statistics, engineering, programming, and business.

Personal characteristics of the CHOLERIC

They are strong-willed, independent, self-sufficient and eager to express themselves before a group if they have some purpose in view. They are insistent upon the acceptance of their ideas or plans, impetuous and impulsive, self-confident and self-reliant.

Choleric Diseases/Conditions

Excessive thirst, irritation of the liver, rough facial skin, yellowing of the eyes, turbidity of the urine, nervousness, upset stomach, bitterness, loss of appetite, nausea, headache, black eyes, dizziness, dry skin, cracked skin on hands and feet, a hot body or fever, boiling pyloric orifice, terrifying dreams, scalp scaling (scalp dandruff), white or brown spots on the face or other parts of the body, hair loss, interest in drinking and eating ice water, constipation.

Foods	Compatible	Inconsistent
VEGGIES	Mushroom, green beans, spinach, lettuce, okra, fava beans, endive, zucchini, potato, wakame, cucumber, tomato, butternut squash, endive, Sweet potato, peas, orach	Ginger, bitter melon, aloe vera, chives, bell pepper, green pepper, eggplant, onion, scallion, radish, shallots, garlic, daikon, asparagus, red cabbage, cabbage, broccoli, cauliflower, artichoke, rhubarb, leeks, celery
FRUITS	Watermelon, orange, tangerine, plum, grapefruit, citrus orange, lime, lemon, kiwi, pomegranate, peach, apricot, figs, persica, ziziphus, nectarine	Apple, grapes, melons, walnuts, hazelnuts, pistachios, dates, coconut, raisin
HERBS	Chicory, purslane, flixweed seeds, chia	Basil, parsley, mint, dill, tarragon, lavender, Angelica, watercress, fenugreek, flaxseed, thyme, rosemary, fennel, oregano, ajwain seeds, cumin, sativa, savory, cress
GRAINS CEREALS	Barley, mung beans, lentils, barley, rice	Split pea, peas, black pea, red lentil (dhal), wheat
NUTS	Pumpkin seeds	Cashew, walnut, pistachios, hazelnut
OILS		Sunflower oil, butter, sesame oil
DRINKS	Doogh, beer, sour pomegranate juice, syrup rhubarb, syrup barberry	
SPICES	Tamarind	Black & white pepper, paprika, curry, fennel, vanilla, celery seeds, cumin, cacao, cloves, cardamom, cinnamon, black
OTHER		Honey, mustard

PHLEGMATIC

Introduction and General Considerations

A person whose constitution tended to have a preponderance of phlegm had a phlegmatic disposition. In the complex elaboration of humorist theory, it was associated with "Water" from the Four Elements of the Universe, the season of Winter, the spleen as the originating organ and Cold and Moist as related qualities. In astrology it showed the influence of the Moon and the planet Venus.

The Phlegmatic Temperament is dominated by the Water element and its basic qualities of Cold and Wet. It is also dominated by the Phlegmatic Humor, which is an umbrella term for all the watery, clear fluids of the body – not just phlegm and mucus, but also plasma, lymph, interstitial fluid, cerebrospinal fluid and synovial fluid (sometimes called the Lymphatic Temperament, since lymph is a very important serous fluid.) Phlegm is the most indolent and passive of all the Four Humors, being Cold and Wet in its basic qualities, and will spontaneously become excessive and aggravated whenever the body is invaded by Cold-natured pathogenic factors, or when the digestive and metabolic fires of the body get too low. Being so passive and indolent in nature, phlegm can linger in the body for a long time, and while it is there, it can impede or obstruct many vital processes, such as digestion, respiration, circulation, etc...

Although the Phlegmatic Humor is generated in the stomach, mainly through a cold and deficient fire of pepsin, one of its main secondary accumulation sites is in the lungs and respiratory tract, and in the head and sinuses. The primary way one can deal with morbid excesses and aggravations of phlegm is to change his dietary habits to stop eating foods that aggravate phlegm. Secondly, one can use herbs, medicinal substances and therapies that are heating and drying in nature to dissolve, concoct, and expel phlegm through the power of contraries.

Personal characteristics of the PHLEGMATIC

They tend to be slow in movement, reserved and distant, deliberative and slow in making decisions. They are typically indifferent to external affairs and have a marked tendency to persevere. Their mood usually stays constant.

Food	Compatible	Inconsistent
VEGGIES	Ginger, bitter melon, aloe vera, leeks, chives, bell pepper, green pepper, eggplant, onion, scallion, radish, celery shallots, garlic, daikon, asparagus, red cabbage, cabbage, broccoli, cauliflower, artichoke, rhubarb	Mushroom, green beans, spinach, lettuce, okra, fava beans, endive, zucchini, potato, wakame, lotusroot cucumber, tomato, butternut squash, endive, sweet potato, peas, orach
FRUITS	Apple, Grapes, melons, walnuts, hazelnuts, pistachios, dates, coconut, raisin, date	Watermelon, orange, kiwi tangerine, plum, pitaya, lemon, grapefruit, citrus orange, lime, jujube, strawberry, pomegranate, peach, apricot, figs, apricot, nectarine, cherry
HERBS	Basil, parsley, mint, dill, satureja tarragon, lavender, angelica, watercress, fenugreek, flaxseed, thyme, rosemary, fennel, oregano, ajwain seeds, cumin, sativa, savory, cress, ginseng, astringent, licorice, fenugreek seeds	Chicory, purslane, flixweed seeds, chia
GRAINS	Split pea, Peas, black peas, red lentil	Barley, mung beans, lentils
NUTS	Cashew, walnut, pistachios, hazelnut,	Pumpkin seeds,
CEREALS	Wheat, rice	Barley
DAIRY	Cheese (salted with walnuts)	Whey, milk, yogurt, cheese
OILS	Sunflower oil, butter, sesame oil	vegetable butter
DRINKS		Doogh, beer,
SPICES	Black & white pepper, fennel, celery seeds, cumin, cacao, cardamom, vanilla, black cumin, laurel, nutmeg, mustard, turmeric, saffron, cloves, curry leaves, vanilla, paprika, Eucalyptus, cinnamon, curry	Tamarind
OTHER	Honey, mustard	

Phlegmatic diseases/conditions

Cause of tumors, of chlorosis, of rheumatism, and cacothymia, arthritis, rheumatoid disease, multiple sclerosis (MS), slow digestion of food, sour rash, fatigue, water flowing from the mouth, Lean nose, low senses, a lot of urine, elimination of urine with high pressure and high volume, weakness and lethargy, grey hair, hair loss and premature aging, stomach pain and back pain, muscle cramps and back pain, neck pain, leg pain, gout, paralysis, potential twisted mouth and face, temblor (Parkinson), weakness of the bladder, dry mouth, white spots on the eyes, poor vision, trouble breathing, palpitations, production of gourd worms or worms at the end of the large intestine.

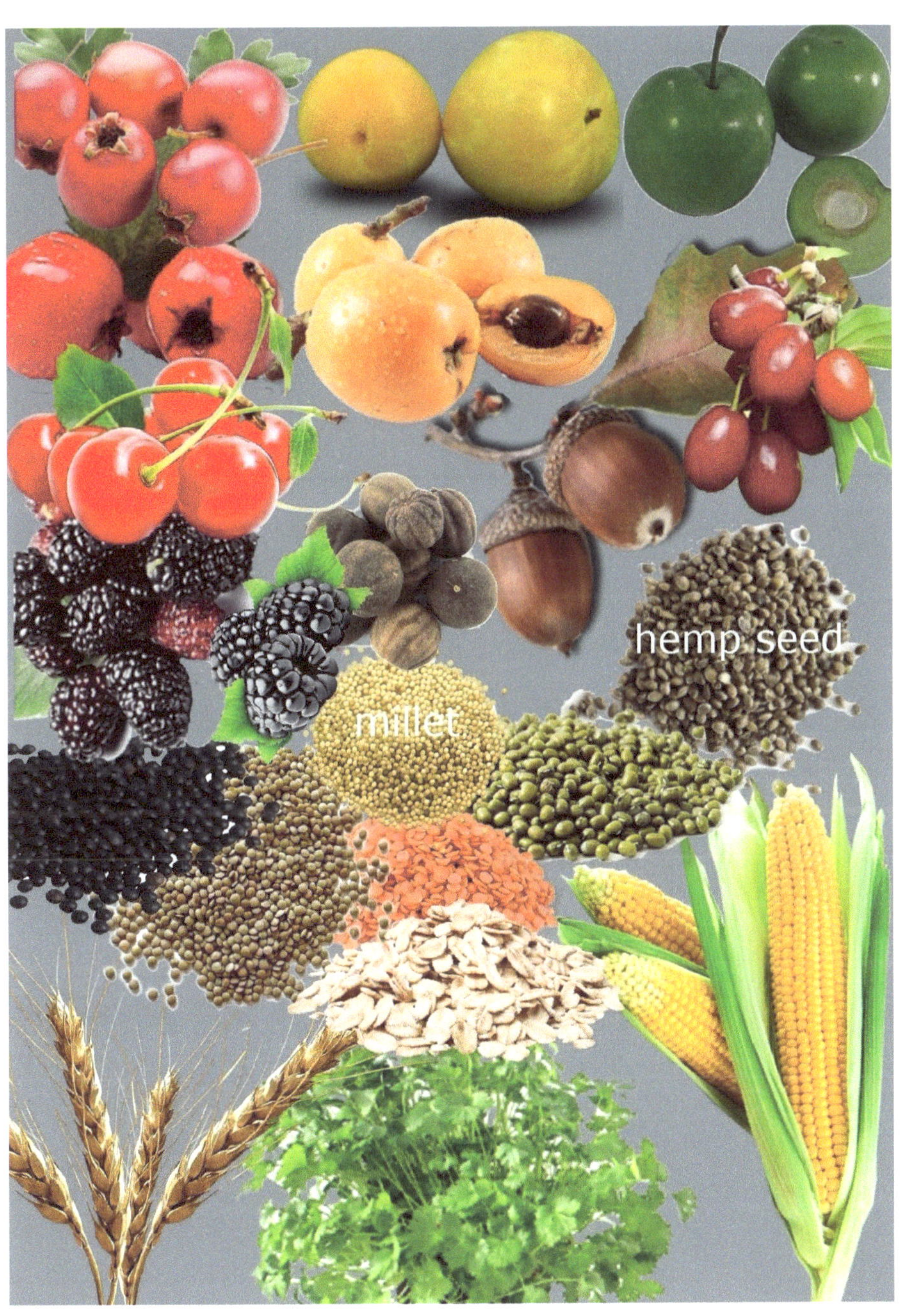
hemp seed
millet

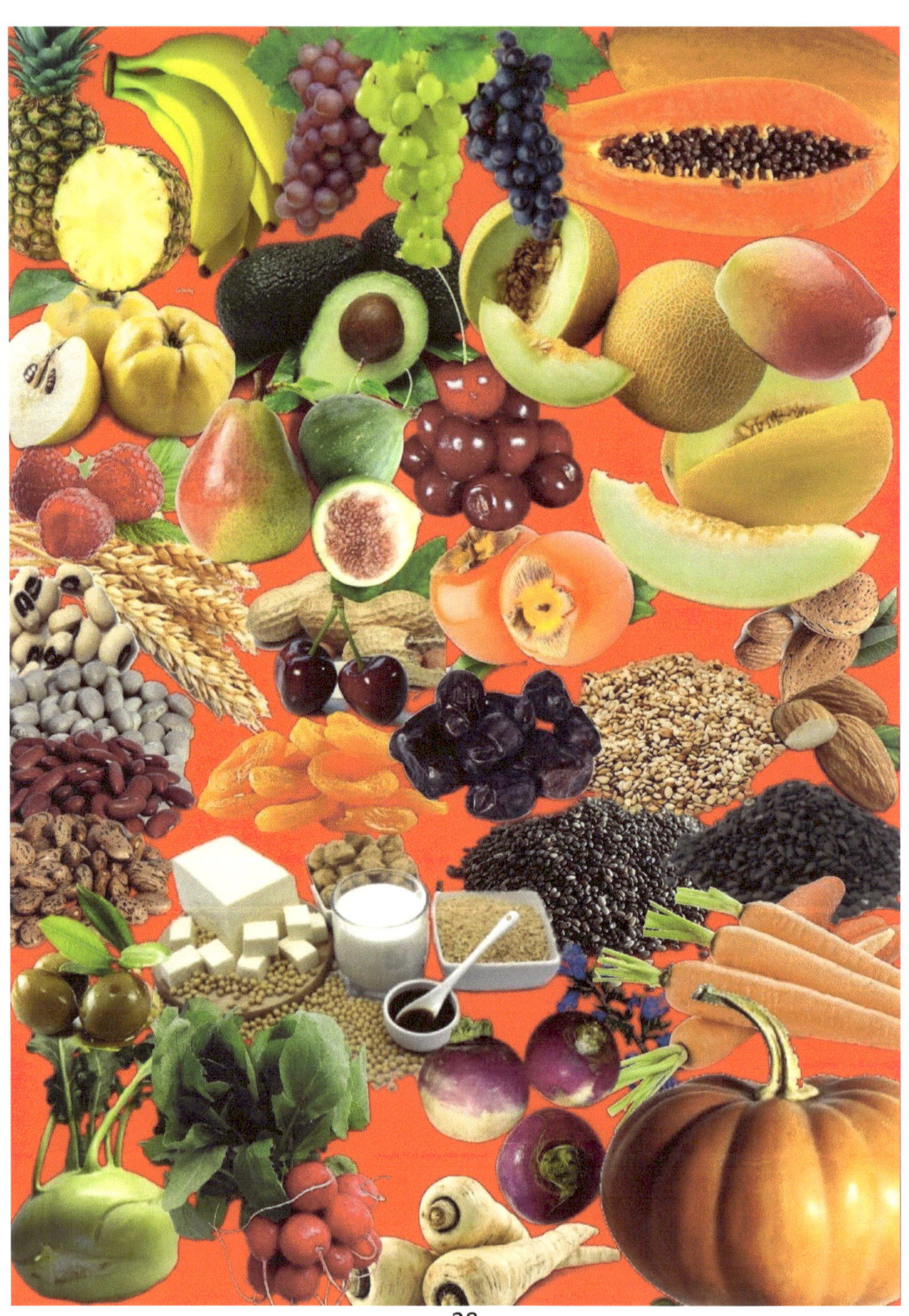

CHOLERIC

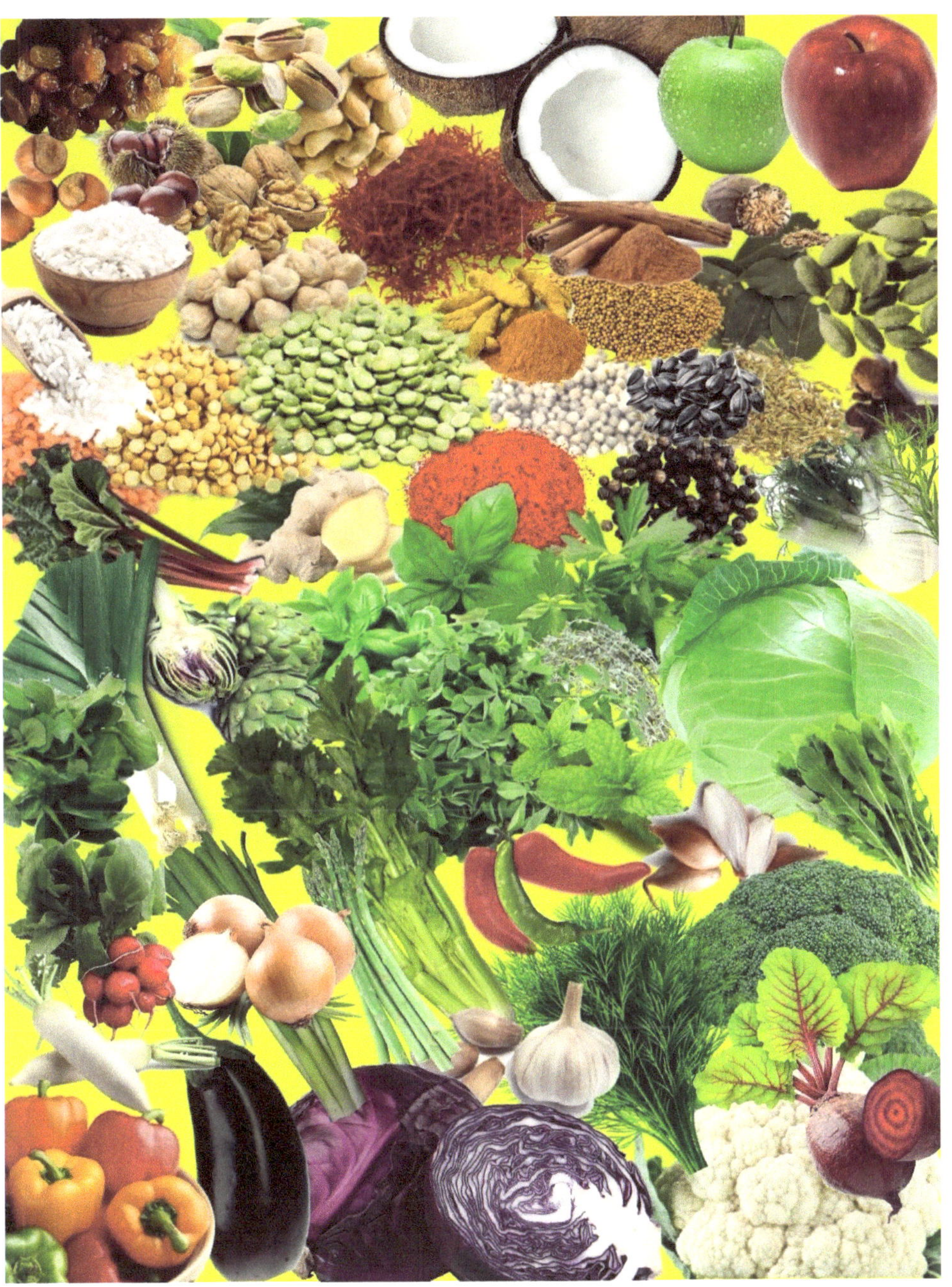

PHLEGMATIC

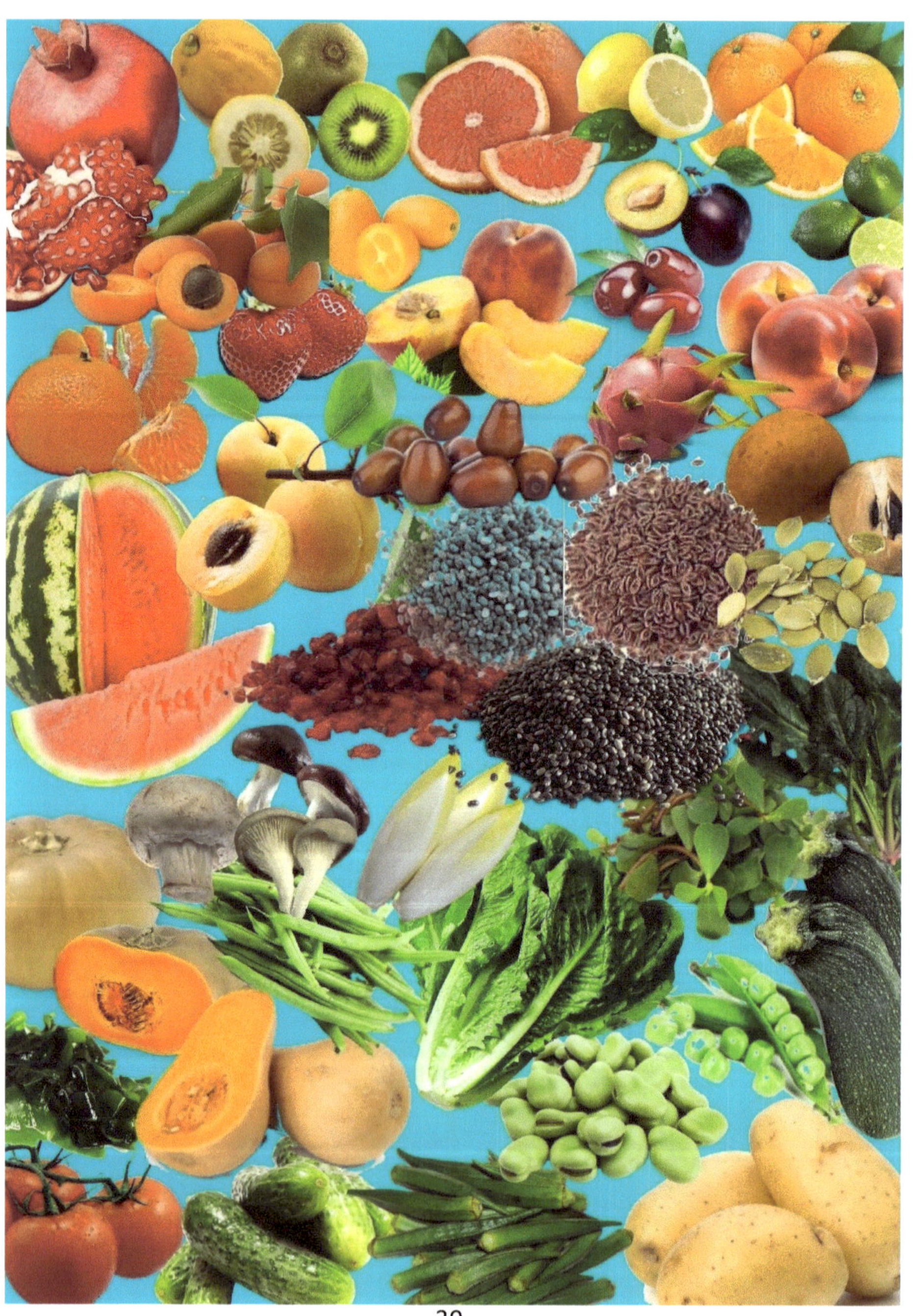

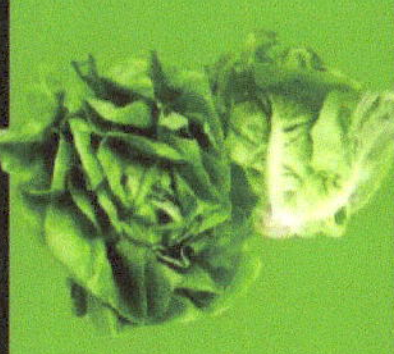
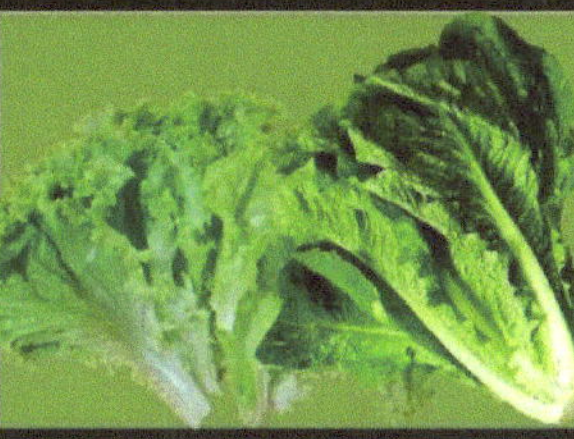
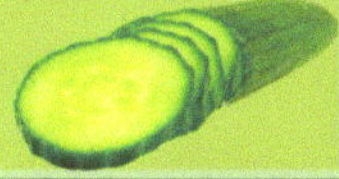

Lettuce

Helps to prevent growth of cancerous cella in body

Anti-Inflammatory

Lowers risk of high blood pressure and heart diseases

Beneficial in reducing risk of diabetes

Controls Anxiety

Qualities
Cold & Moist

Vitamin
A, C, K, manganese

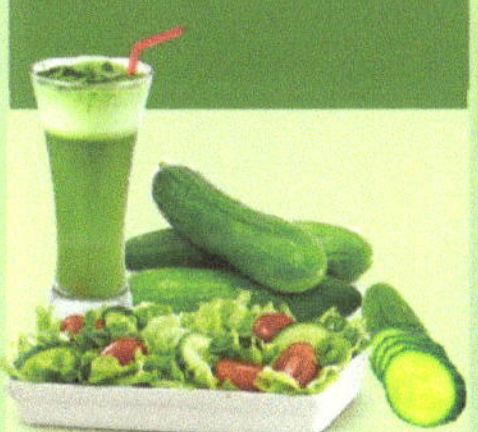
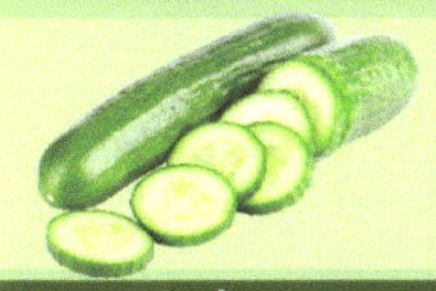
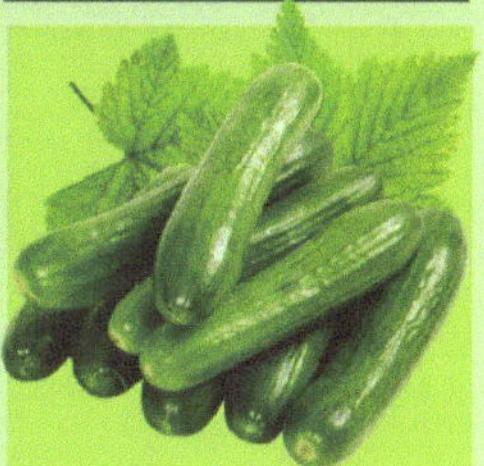

Cucumber

Helps lower blood pressure

Provides bright & glowing complexion

Keep body healthy & functioning

Aids in managing diabetes

Qualities
Cold & Moist

Helps prevent constipation

Vitamin
A, B, C
magnesium potassium

Prevents constipation and keeps kidneys healthy

Vitamin

C, A
B1

reduce the risk of developing prostate cancer and colon cancer

Healthy sleep

relieve excess flatulence and stomach discomfort

Grapefruit

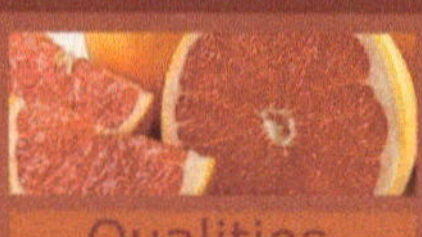

Qualities
Cold & Moist

reduce the burning sensation that arises during fever

help to regulate the flow of sugar in diabetics

help to quench thirst

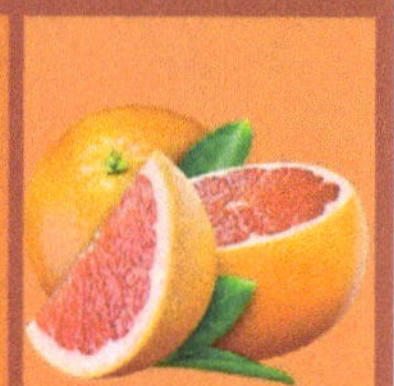

useful for solving the problem of indigestion

Reduce inflammation

Strawberries

Reduce risk of eye related ailments

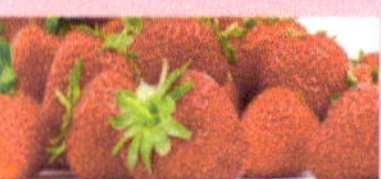

Help maintain normal blood pressure

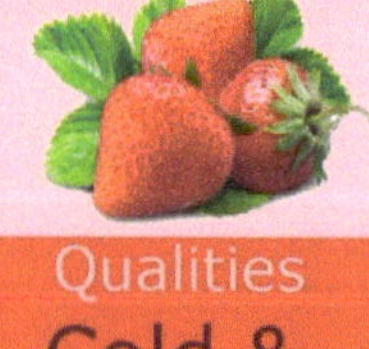

vitamin

B6,C
E, K

Boost immune System

Qualities
Cold & Moist

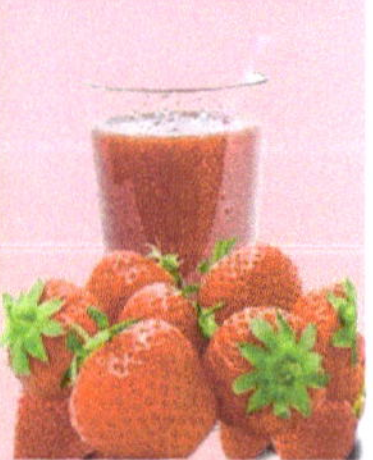

Help regulate proper functioning of nervous system

Lower risk of arthritis, gout and cancer

Prevent heart disease and reduce cholesterol

Pomegranates

help to reduce the effects of dental plaque and protect against various oral diseases

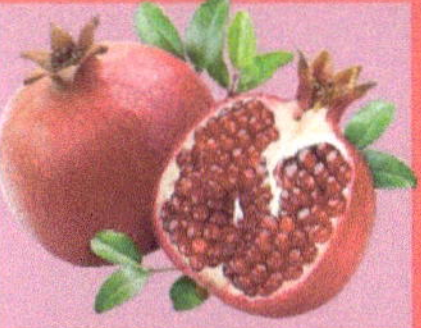

reduce the risk of developing cancer

Vitamin

A, C, E

Help to reduce symptoms of anemia, including exhaustion, dizziness, weakness, and hearing loss

Pomegranates

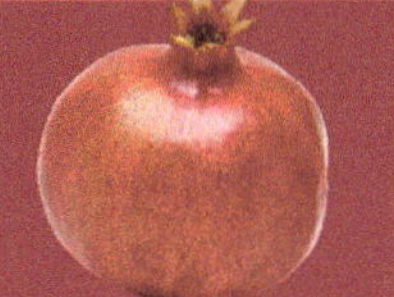

Qualities
Cold & Moist

Alleviate the symptoms of gastric ulcers

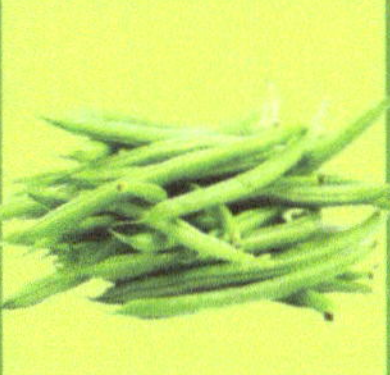

have anti-oxidant, anti-viral and anti-tumor properties

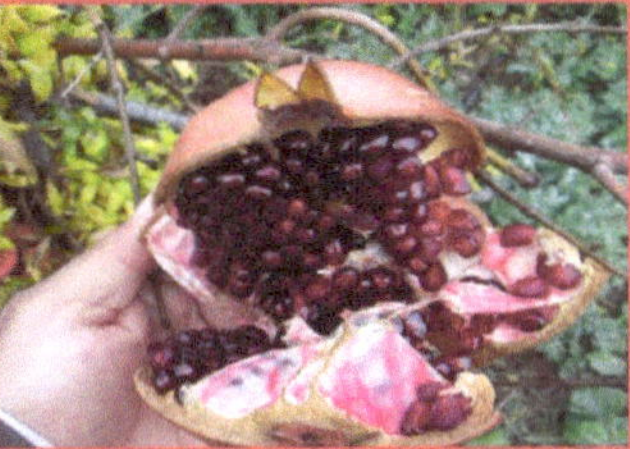

help in maintaining a smooth and wrinkle_free skin

Boost heart health

Green Beans

Help to prevent colon cancer

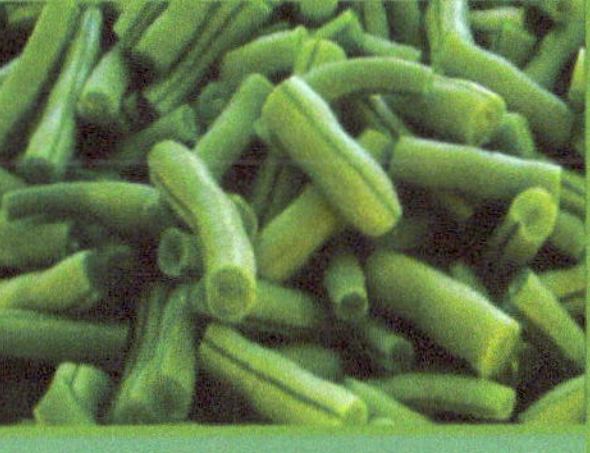

Boost immune system

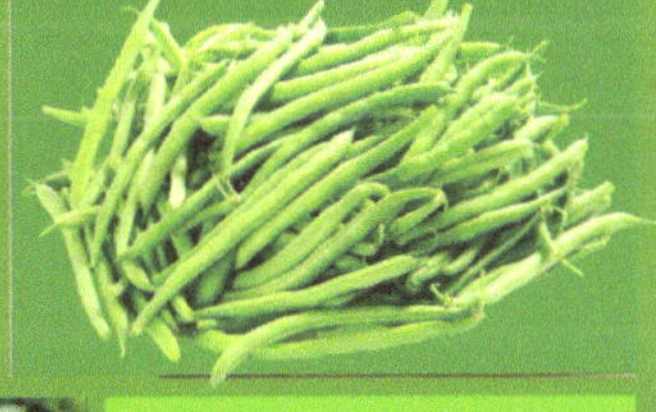

Eye Health and Bone Health

Green Beans

Aid in managing diabetes

Qualities
Cold & Moist

help reduce the risk of heart disease

Vitamin

A, K
silicon

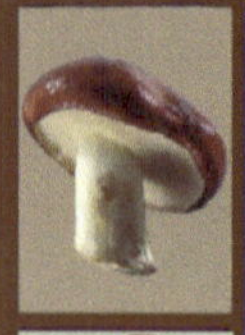
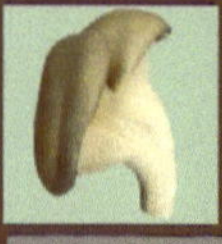

relief from prostate cancer and diabetes

Mushroom

helps in weight loss

strengthens bones and teeth

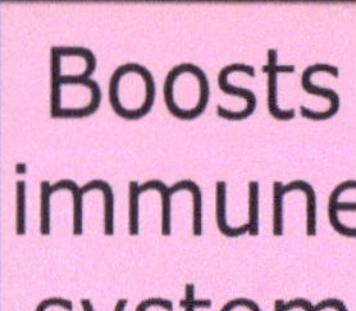

Boosts immune system

relief from high cholesterol levels, breast cancer

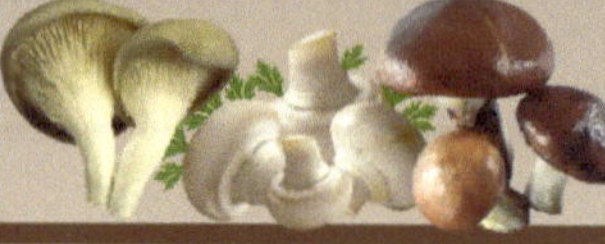

Vitamin D
Riboflavin
Copper

Blood sugar: Regulates sugar absorption in diabetics and prevents heart disease

Scurvy:
Rich in vitamin C

Healing:
Gives relief from eye infection, nausea, arthritis, gout, fever and congestion

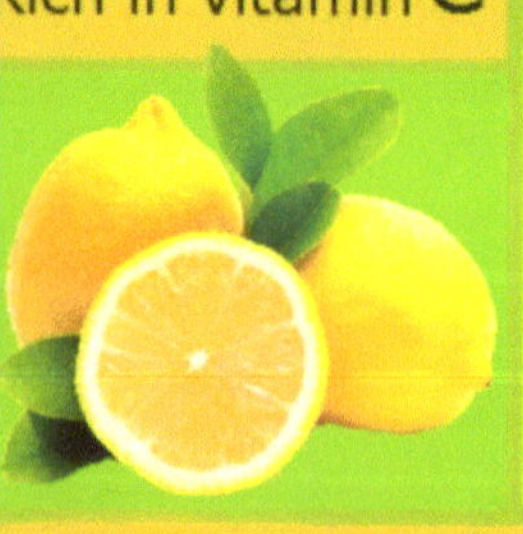

Digestion:
Stimulates digestive system

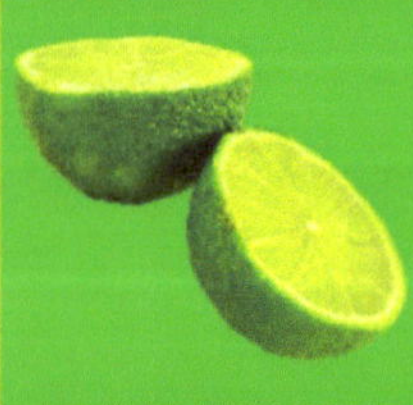

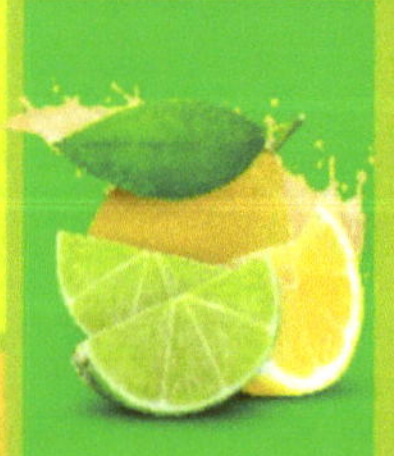

Weight loss

Lime

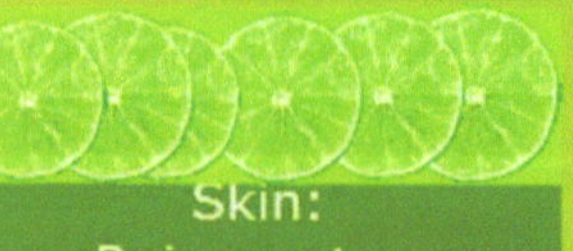

Hair:
Help to eliminate dandruff from hair follicles

Qualities
Cold & Moist

Skin:
Rejuvenates, protects from infection and reduces body odor

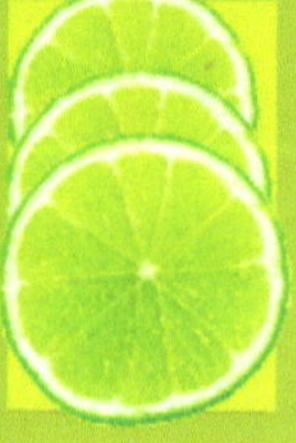

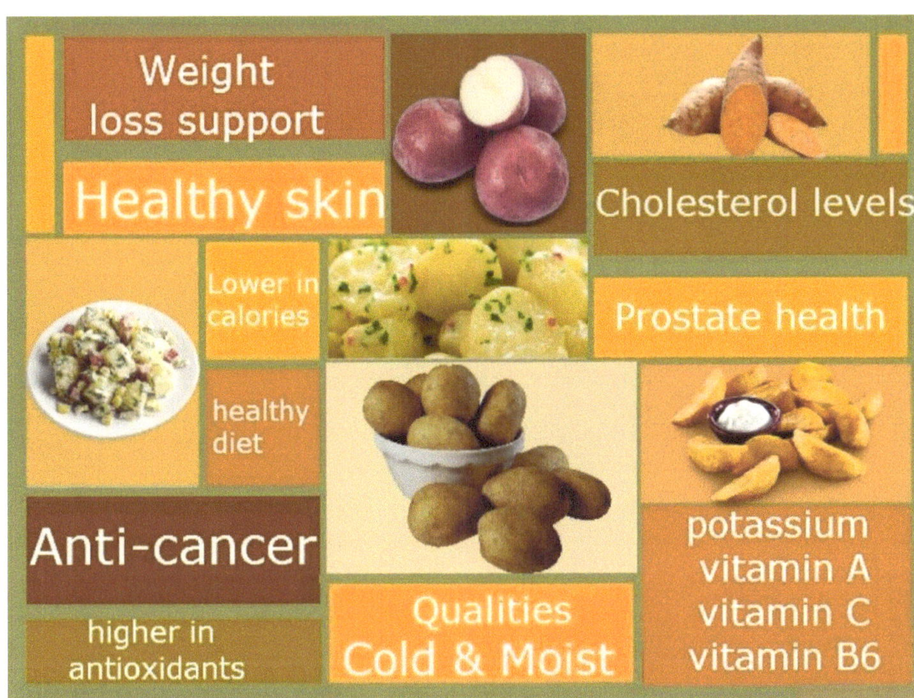

Weight loss support
Healthy skin
Cholesterol levels
Lower in calories
Prostate health
healthy diet
Anti-cancer
higher in antioxidants
Qualities
Cold & Moist
potassium
vitamin A
vitamin C
vitamin B6

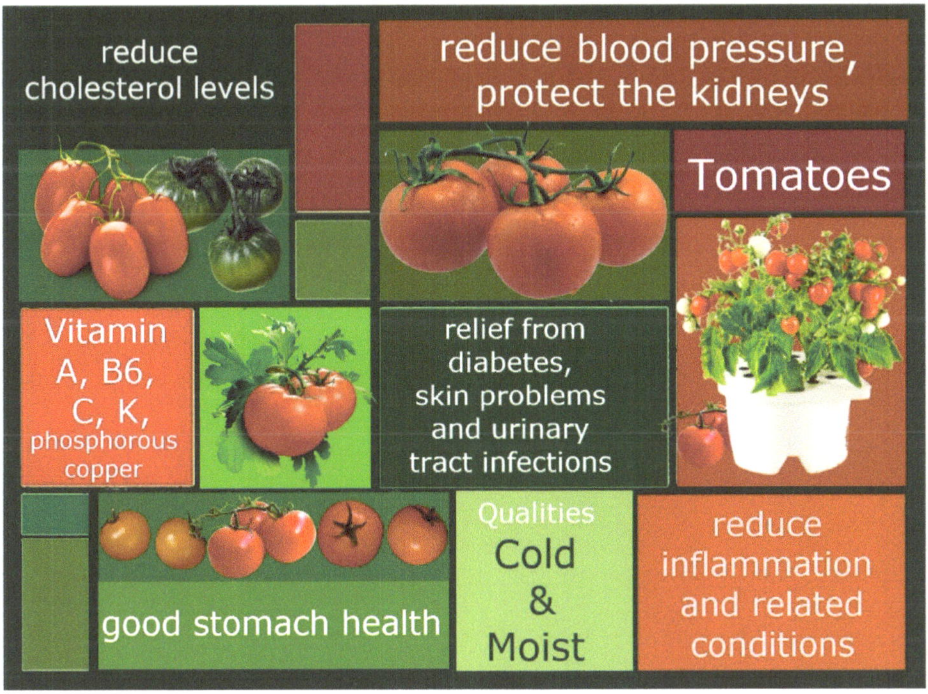

reduce cholesterol levels
reduce blood pressure, protect the kidneys
Tomatoes
Vitamin A, B6, C, K, phosphorous copper
relief from diabetes, skin problems and urinary tract infections
good stomach health
Qualities
Cold & Moist
reduce inflammation and related conditions

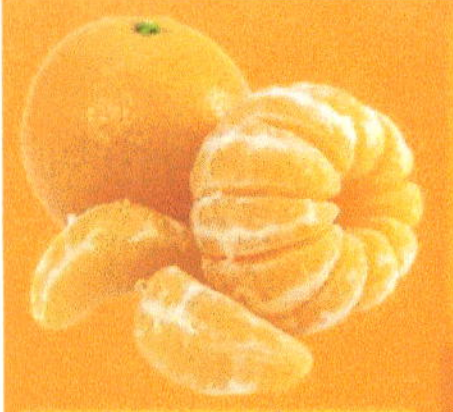

help lower blood sugar levels

boost heart health
lower the risk of disease
reduce liver cancer

help reduce the risk of cataracts and improve night vision

Vitamin

A
B1
C

Orange

Qualities
Cold & Moist

Prevent cancer such as skin, lung, breast, stomach, and colon

help lower cholesterol levels

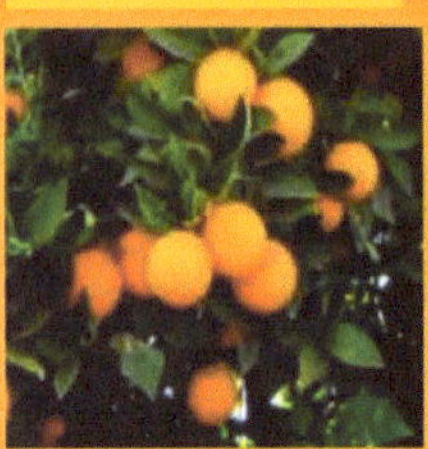

prevent kidney disease and reduce the risk of kidney stones

Helps to lower total cholesterol levels

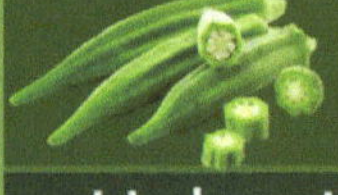

Okra

Boosts immune system

Helps to relax blood vessels and arteries

Aids in improving digestion

Qualities

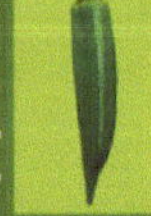

Cold & Most

Reduces appearance of scars, acne and wrinkles

protects heart health

Vitamin
A, B, C,
E, K

calcium
iron
magnesium
potassium

Protects eyes against cataracts and macular degeneration

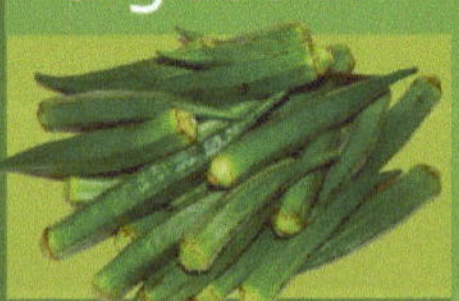

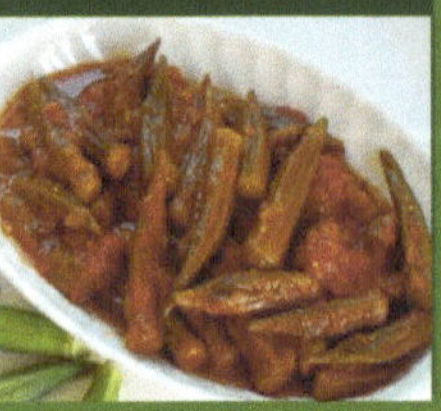

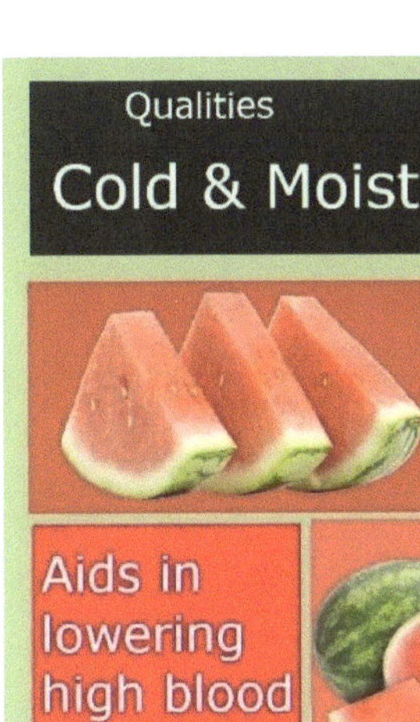
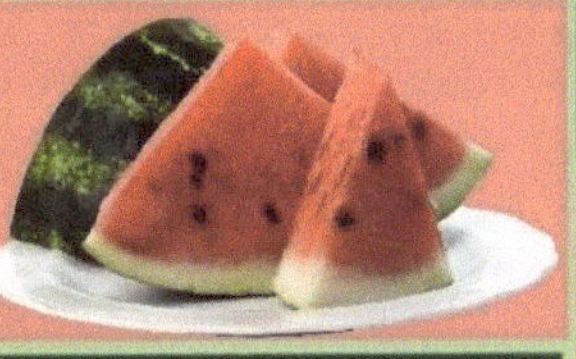

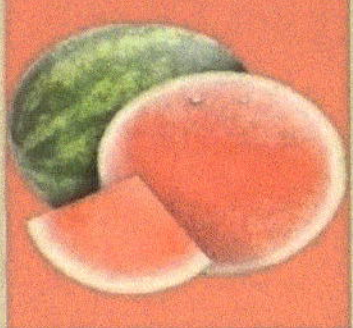

Qualities
Cold & Moist
Helps prevent heat stroke & cancer
Watermelon
Aids in lowering high blood pressure
Beneficial in curing erectile dysfunction
Reduces risk of kidney disorders
Vitamin A, B6, C
calcium magnesium
Helps lower blood sugar levels in diabetics

Prevents age-related macular degeneration
Beneficial for good eyesight
Helps maintain normal blood pressure
Spinach
Provides neurological benefits
Aids in strengthening of muscles
Qualities
Cold & Moist
Vitamin A, B6, C Iron Magnesium Calcium

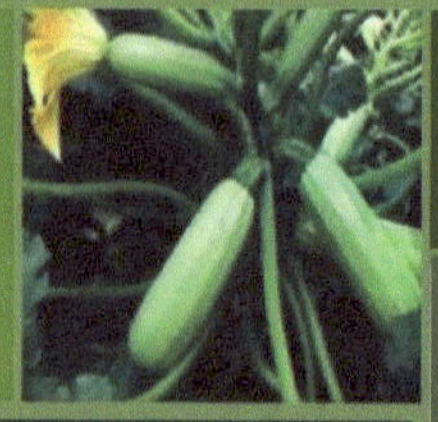
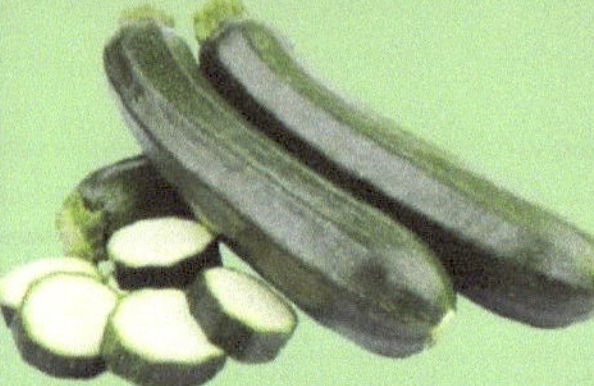

Helps to prevent cancer and cardiovascular diseases
Zucchini
Helps maintain optimal health
Vitamin B1, B2, B6
Omega3 magnesium potassium
Protects against infections and diseases
Beneficial in losing weight
Gives relief from aching symptoms of rheumatoid arthritis
Qualities
Cold & Moist

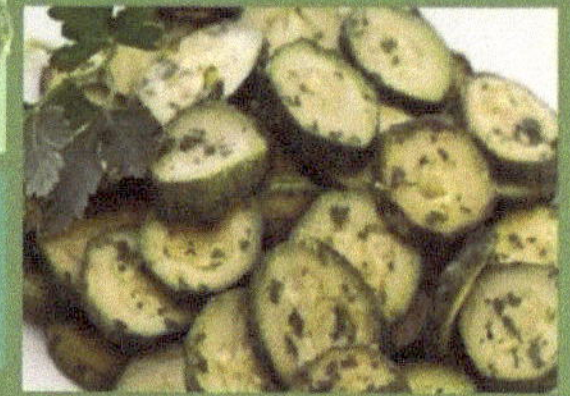
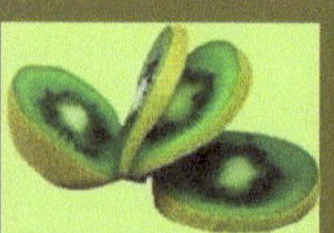
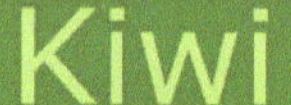
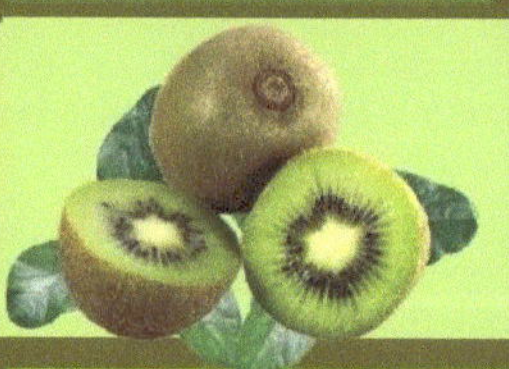
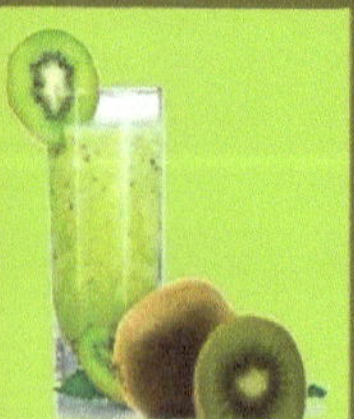

Qualities
Cold & Moist
Kiwi
Rich in antioxidant properties
Vitamin
A
C
E
K
helps to better sleep
Lowers risk of diabetes and cancer
Beneficial for fetal development
Aids in maintaining healthy digestive system

Figs

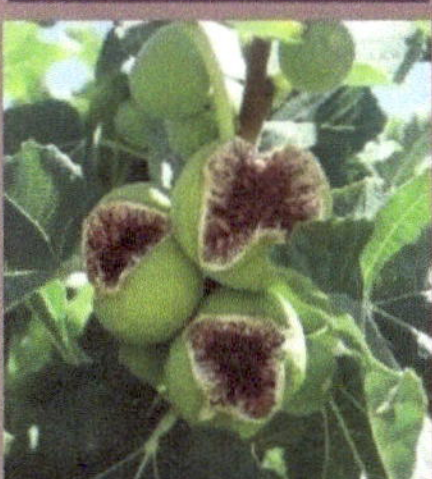

Strengthens Bones

Rich in potassium, regulates sugar absorption in diabetics

Helps to correct sexual dysfunction

Qualities
Warm & Moist

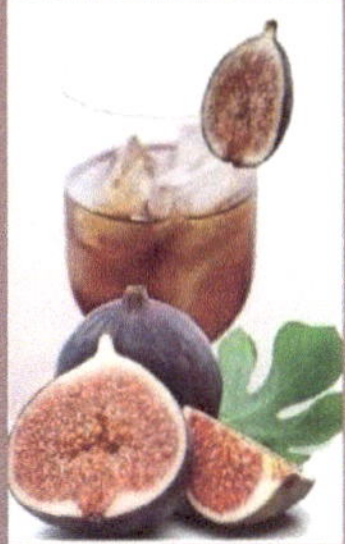

Lowers cholesterol, risk of coronary heart diseases and prevents hypertension

Prevents vision loss caused by macular degeneration

Vitamin
A
B1
B2

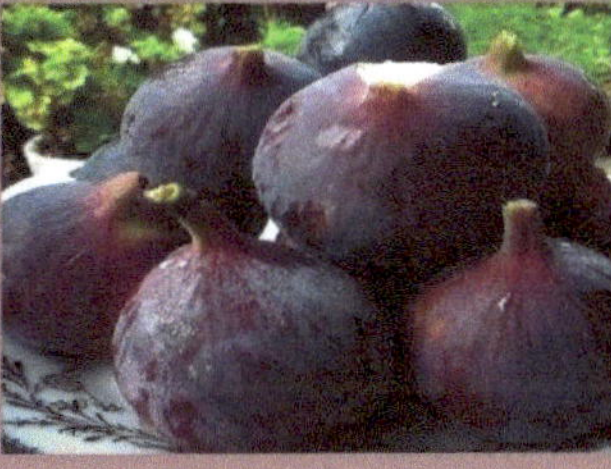

Reduces risk of colon cancer

Turnips

Qualities
Warm & Moist

excellent source of antioxidants

Helps to improve eyesight

Boosts immune system

Aids in weight loss

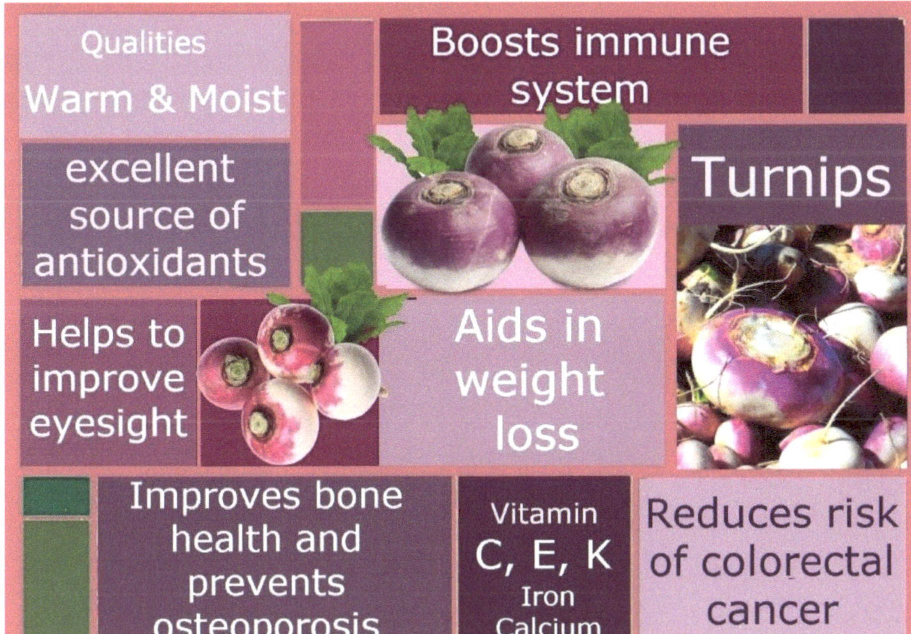

Improves bone health and prevents osteoporosis

Vitamin
C, E, K
Iron
Calcium

Reduces risk of colorectal cancer

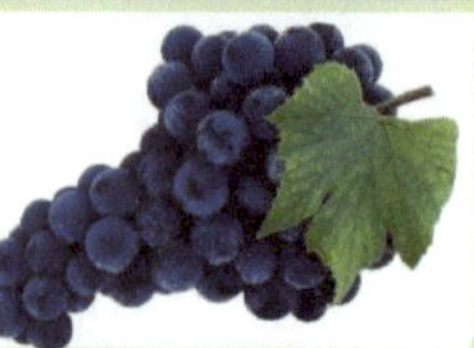

Grapes

Improve brain function and prevent Alzheimer's disease
Boost immune system and prevent fatigue
Reduce risk of kidney diseases
Help cure asthma and migraine
Prevent heart attacks
Qualities
Warm & Moist
Provide relief from constipation and indigestion
Strengthen bones help prevent cavities
Vitamin A, B6, C calcium iron phosphorus

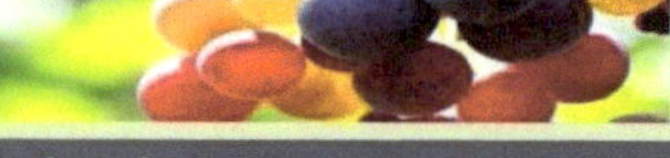

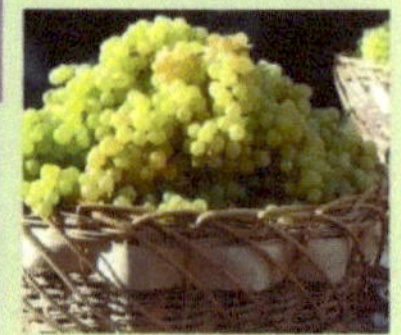

helps to lower cholesterol levels

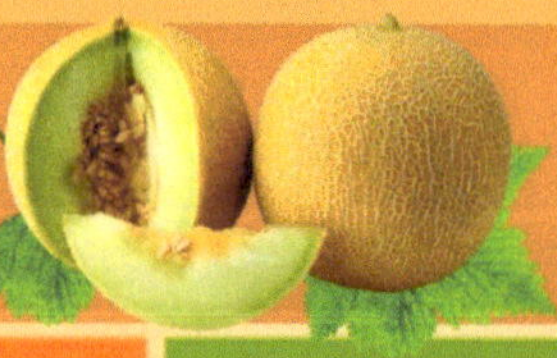

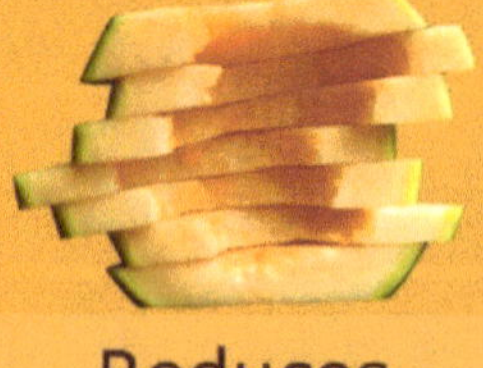

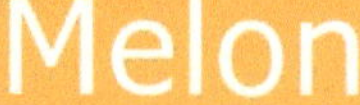

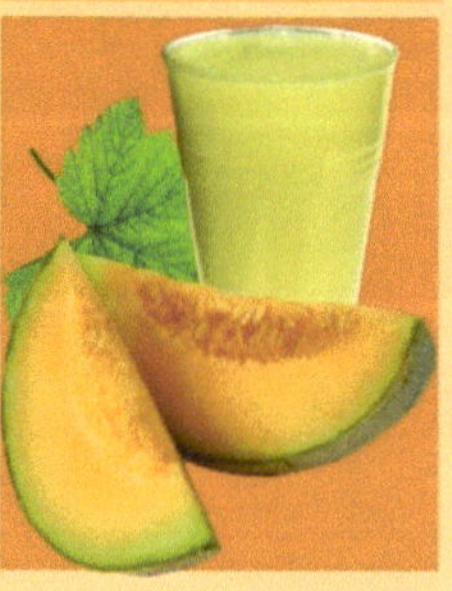

Helps to prevent kidney-related diseases
Qualities
Warm & Moist
Improves insulin metabolism
Prevents arthritis
Boosts immunity and prevents cancer
Melon
Beneficial for healthy eyes
Reduces inflammation
Vitamin A, C, B6

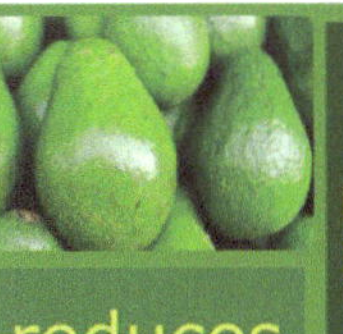

reduces liver damage

helps in maintaining blood sugar levels and has antioxidant properties

Avocado

helps in keeping eyes healthy

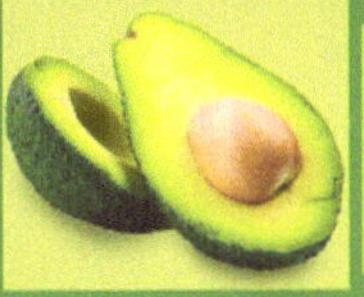

protection from cardiovascular disease and diabetes

Qualities

Warm & Moist

Vitamin A, B6, B-12 C, D, K, E calcium iron copper

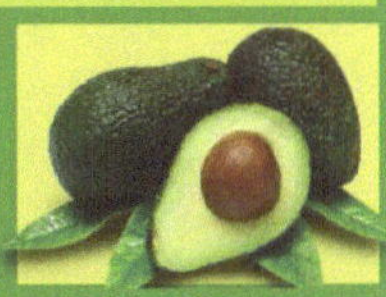

treating osteoarthritis and enhancing the absorption of nutrients for the body

protects the skin from signs of aging and the harmful effects of UV rays

reduces the risk of cancer

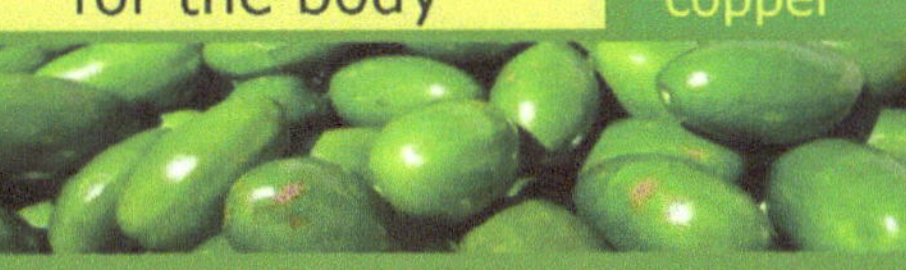

Qualities Warm & moist

improve digestion

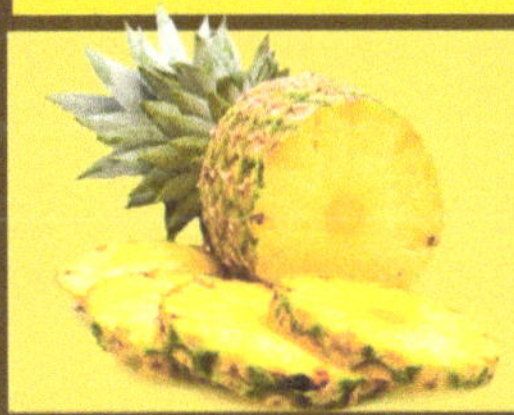

improve the immune system and increase circulation

Pineapples

Vitamin B6, C Potassium Calcium

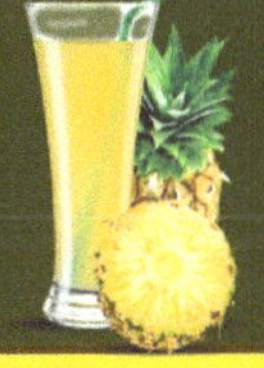

strengthen bones, improve oral health

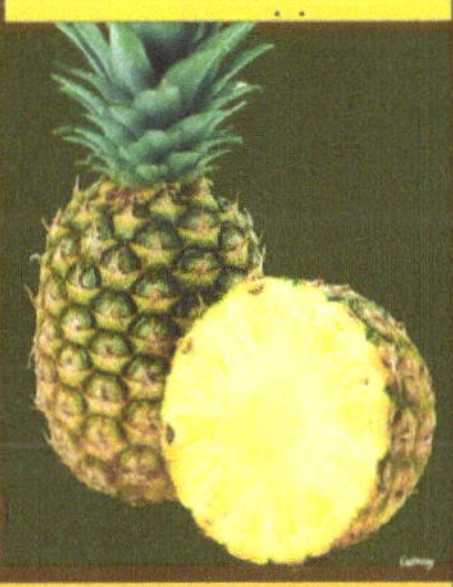

reduce inflammation, prevent cancer, improve heart health

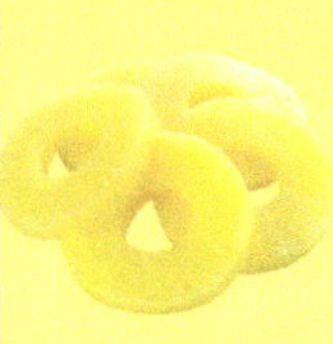

help lose weight

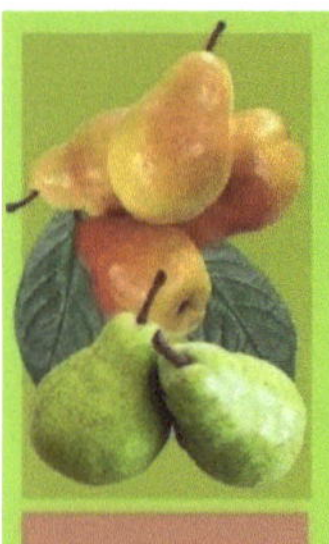

Improved Circulation and Red Blood Cell Count

Qualities
Warm & Moist

Boosts immune system

Vitamin
B
C
K

Treats eczema and dermatitis

Pears

Bone Health

Improves digestion and intestinal health

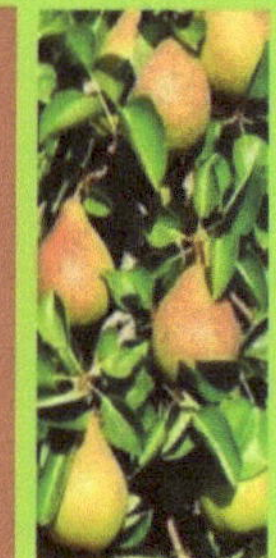

Helps prevent cancer and cardiovascular diseases

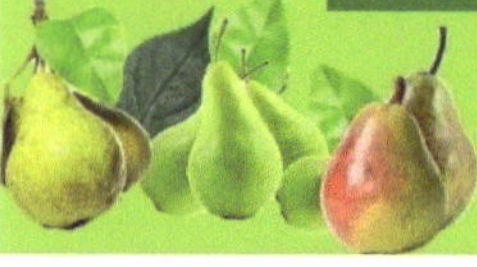

Aids to Skin, Hair, and Eyes

Aids in treating piles & anemia

Banana

Provides relief from stomach ulcers & constipation

Reduces inflammation from arthritis & gout

Keeps eyes & bones healthy

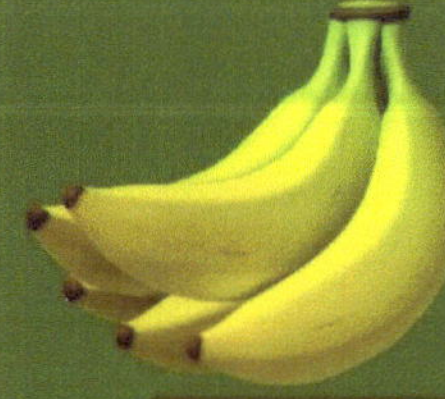

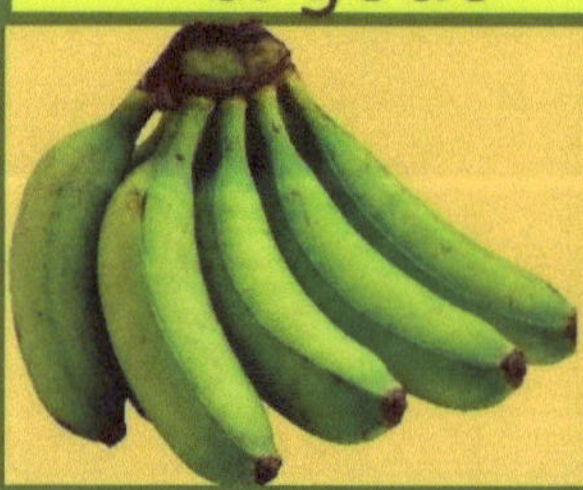

Helps cure kidney disorders

Qualities
Warm & Moist

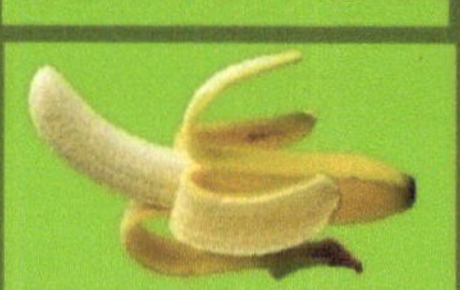

Vitamin
B6, C

fiber
protein

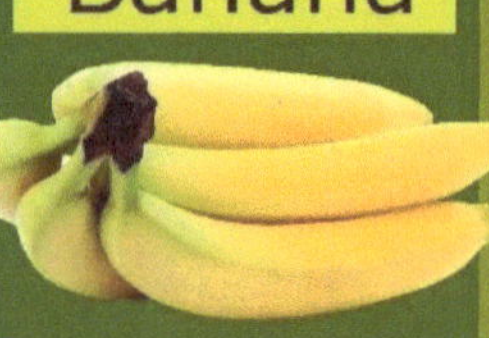

Prevent heart disease

Boost immune system

Carrots

Qualities
Warm & Moist

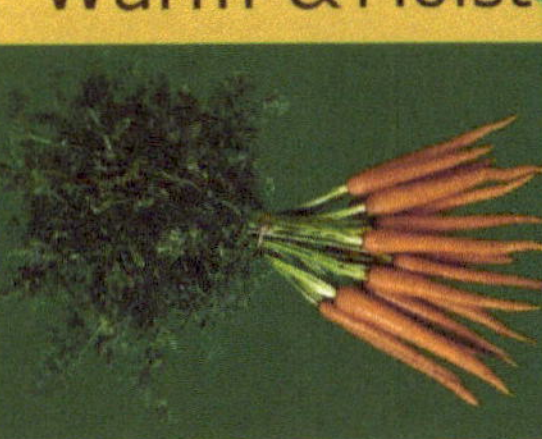

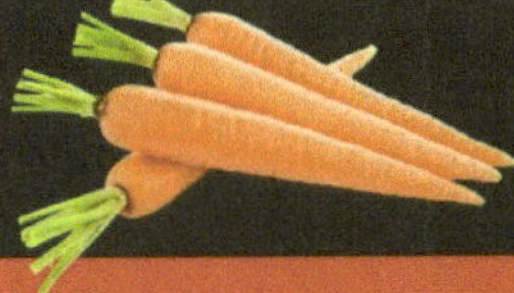

Improve eyesight

Maintain good digestive health

Vitamin A, B8, C, K
iron
copper
manganese

Regulate blood sugar levels

Reduce high blood pressure

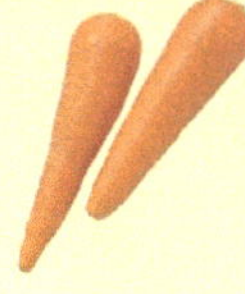

help lose weight, manage diabetes, reduce stress

Eggplant

protect the digestive system

Vitamin B6, C, K
magnesium
phosphorous
copper
potassium
manganese

Qualities
Warm & Dry

reduce symptoms of anemia

protect infants from birth defects, and even prevent cancer

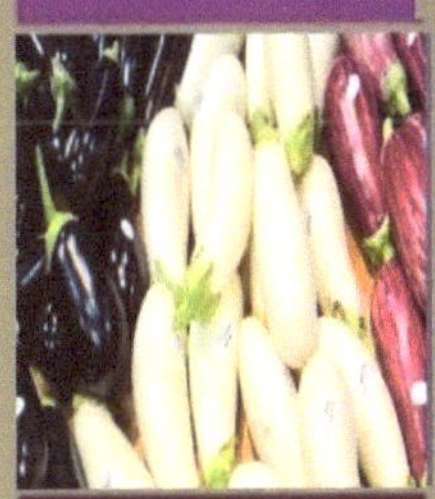

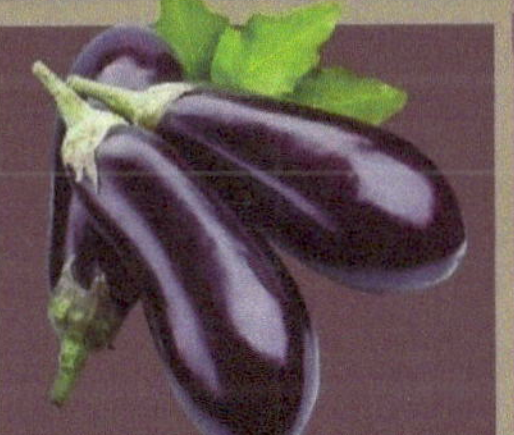

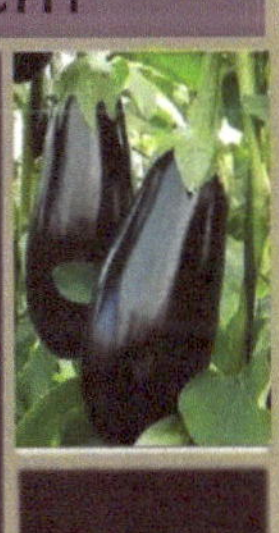

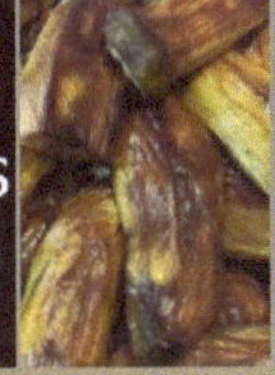

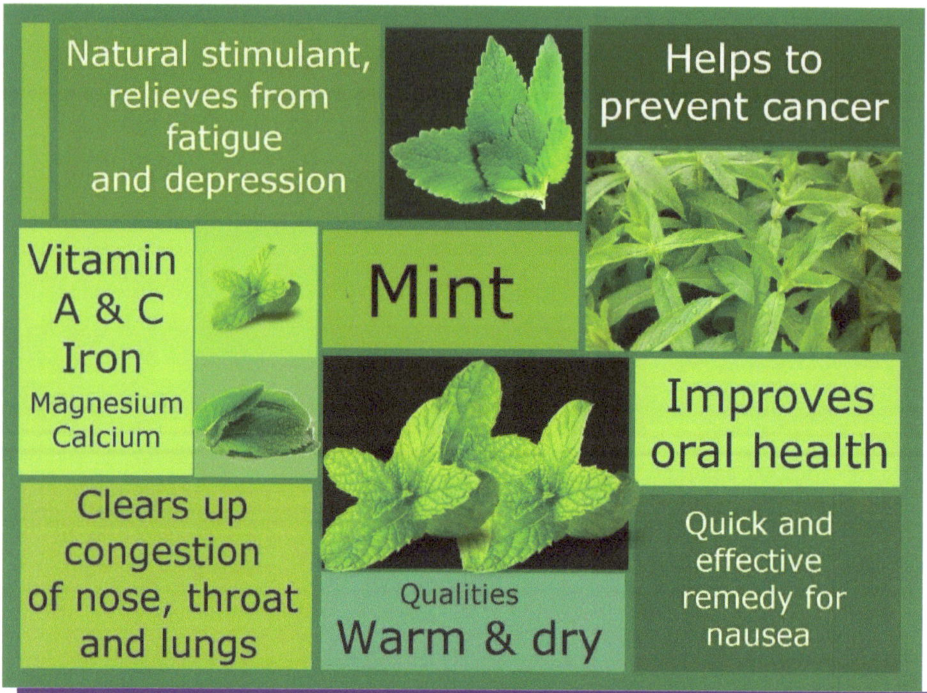

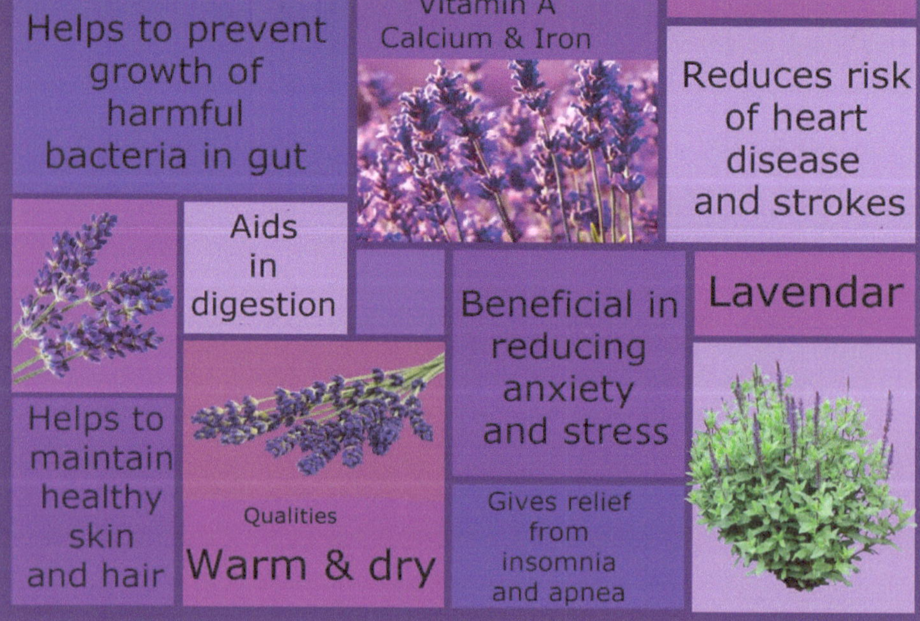

Natural stimulant, relieves from fatigue and depression

Helps to prevent cancer

Vitamin A & C Iron
Magnesium Calcium

Mint

Improves oral health

Clears up congestion of nose, throat and lungs

Qualities
Warm & dry

Quick and effective remedy for nausea

Helps to prevent growth of harmful bacteria in gut

Vitamin A Calcium & Iron

Reduces risk of heart disease and strokes

Aids in digestion

Helps to maintain healthy skin and hair

Beneficial in reducing anxiety and stress

Lavendar

Qualities
Warm & dry

Gives relief from insomnia and apnea

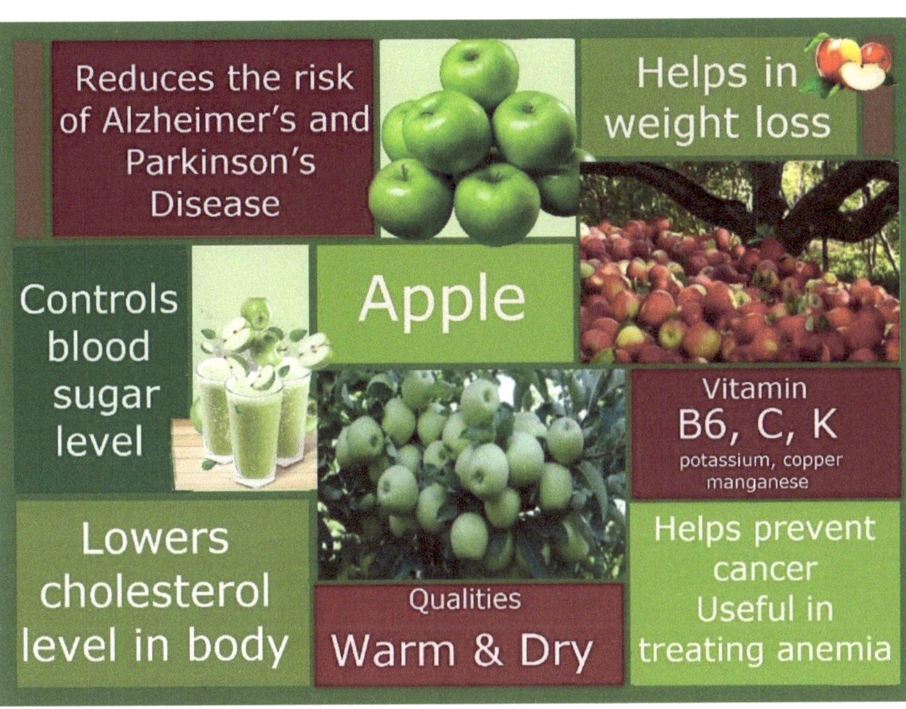

Reduces the risk of Alzheimer's and Parkinson's Disease
Helps in weight loss
Controls blood sugar level
Apple
Vitamin B6, C, K
potassium, copper manganese
Lowers cholesterol level in body
Qualities
Warm & Dry
Helps prevent cancer
Useful in treating anemia

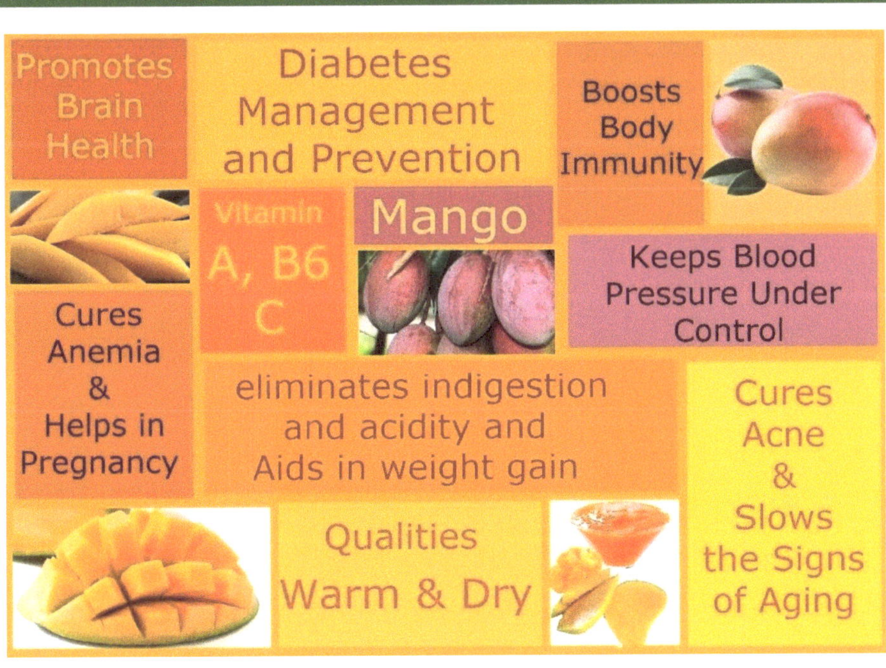

Promotes Brain Health
Diabetes Management and Prevention
Boosts Body Immunity
Vitamin A, B6 C
Mango
Keeps Blood Pressure Under Control
Cures Anemia & Helps in Pregnancy
eliminates indigestion and acidity and Aids in weight gain
Cures Acne & Slows the Signs of Aging
Qualities
Warm & Dry

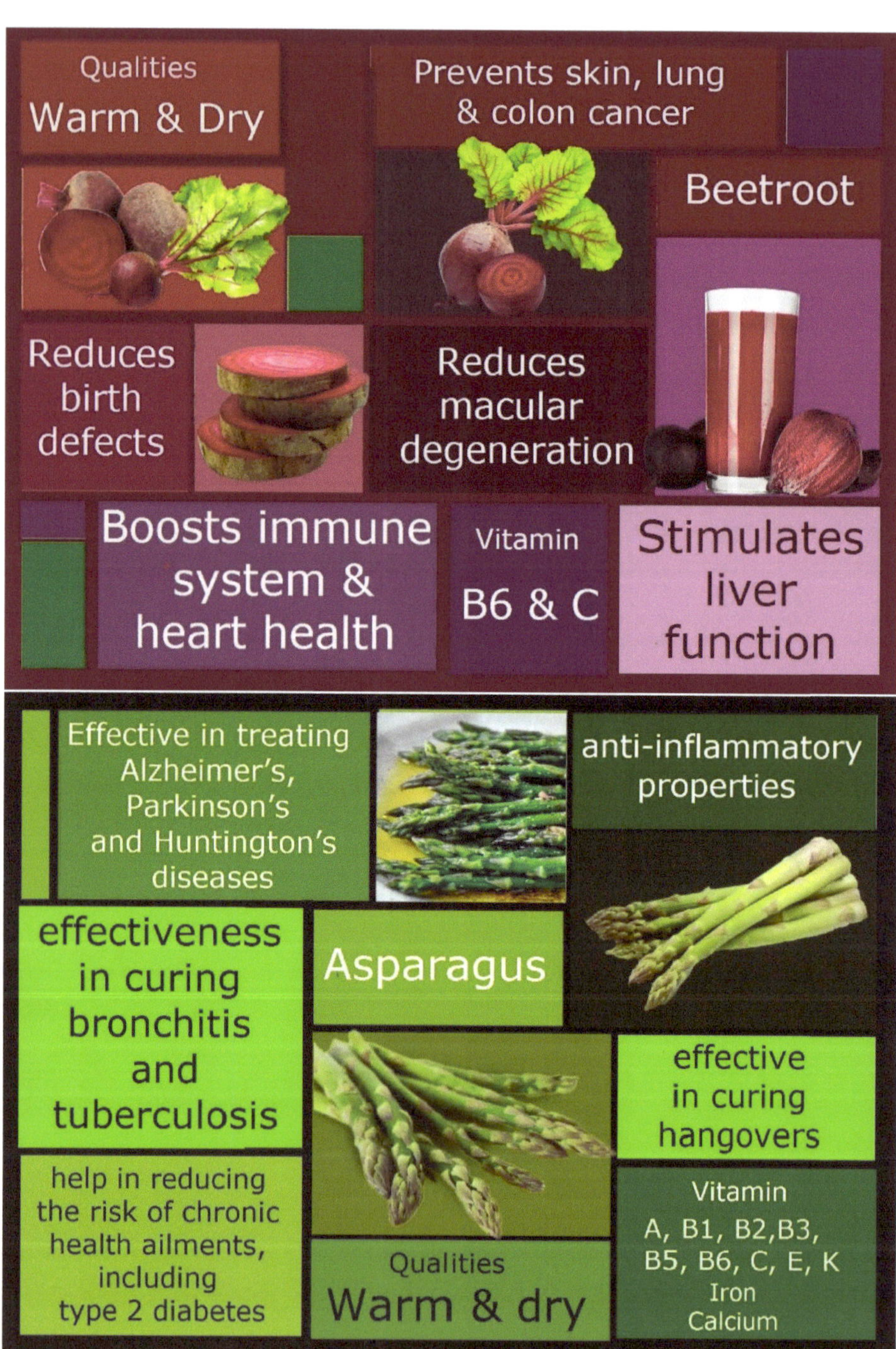

Qualities
Warm & Dry
Prevents skin, lung & colon cancer
Beetroot
Reduces birth defects
Reduces macular degeneration
Boosts immune system & heart health
Vitamin B6 & C
Stimulates liver function
Effective in treating Alzheimer's, Parkinson's and Huntington's diseases
anti-inflammatory properties
effectiveness in curing bronchitis and tuberculosis
Asparagus
effective in curing hangovers
help in reducing the risk of chronic health ailments, including type 2 diabetes
Qualities
Warm & dry
Vitamin A, B1, B2, B3, B5, B6, C, E, K
Iron
Calcium

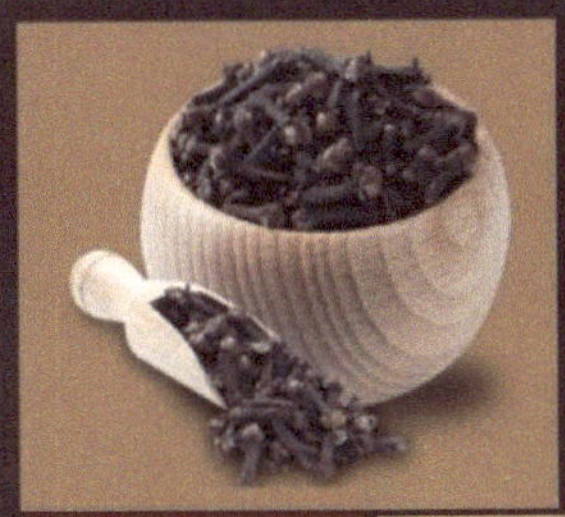
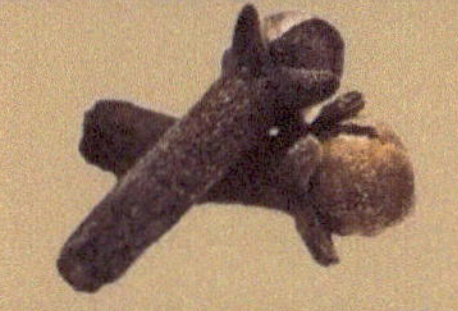
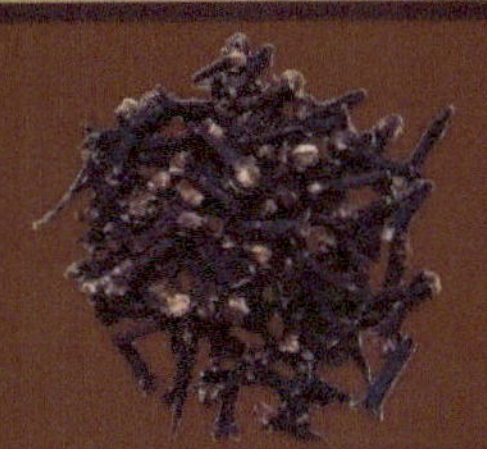
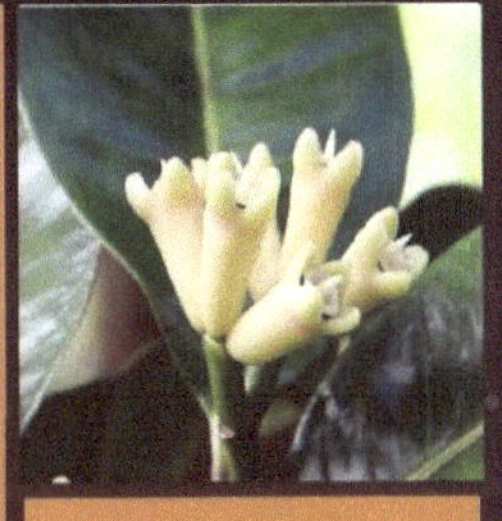

Helps to control blood sugar levels
Aids in digestion
Vitamin
A
B6
B12
D
E
K
Protects liver against infections
Cloves
Qualities
Warm & dry
Protects liver against infections
Gives relief from inflammation & pain

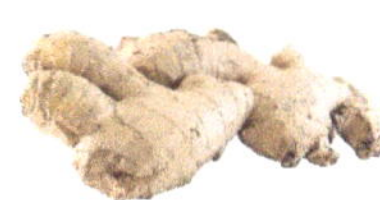
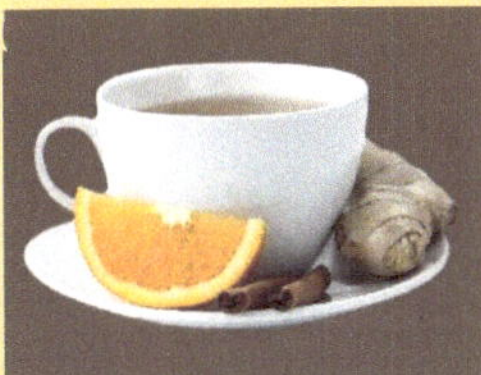
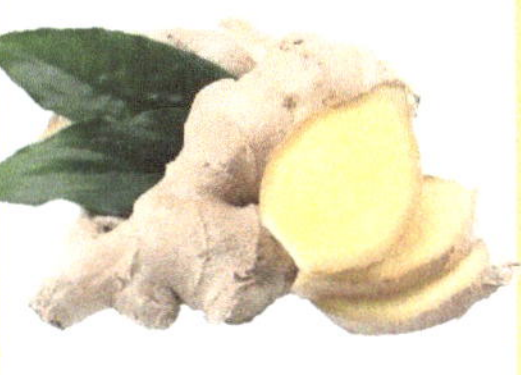

Reduces risk of cancer
Cures diarrhea
Boosts bone health & relieves joint pain
Helps cure nausea
Provides relief from menstrual cramps
Ginger
Regulates high sugar levels
Qualities
Warm & Dry
Facilitates digestion
Builds appetite

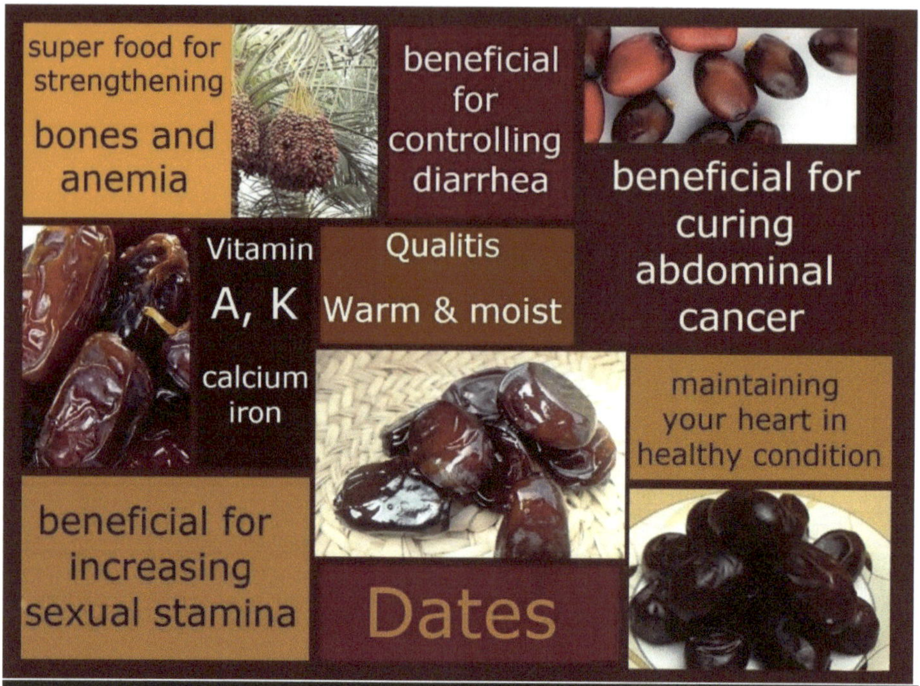

super food for strengthening
bones and anemia
beneficial for controlling diarrhea
beneficial for curing abdominal cancer
Vitamin A, K
calcium iron
Qualitis
Warm & moist
maintaining your heart in healthy condition
beneficial for increasing sexual stamina
Dates

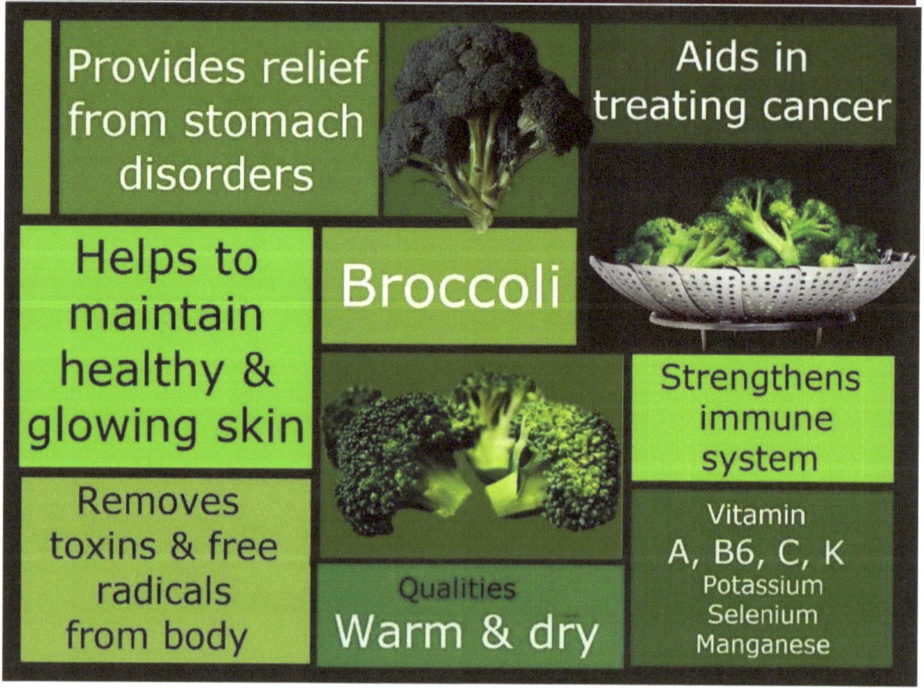

Provides relief from stomach disorders
Aids in treating cancer
Helps to maintain healthy & glowing skin
Broccoli
Strengthens immune system
Removes toxins & free radicals from body
Qualities
Warm & dry
Vitamin A, B6, C, K
Potassium
Selenium
Manganese

Helps to alleviate pain related to arthrits

Bell pepper

Beneficial in preventing diabetes

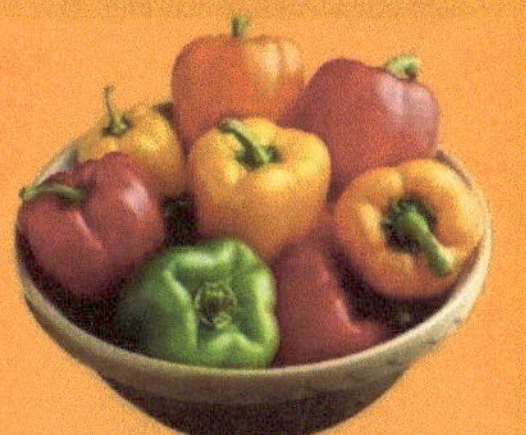

Aids in treating pulmonary hepatic & gastric cancers

Improving bone health

Qualities
Warm & Dry

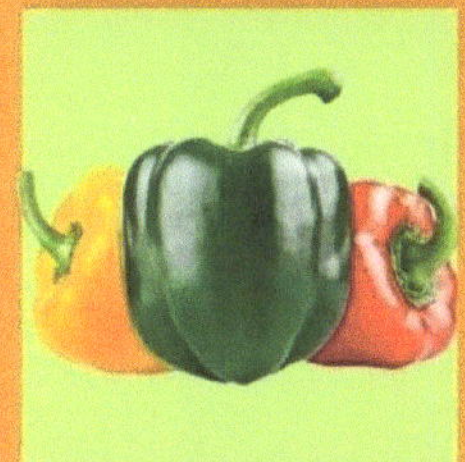

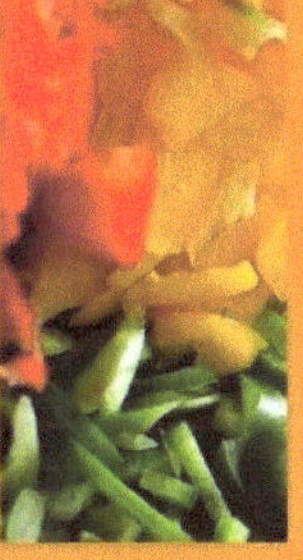

Vitamin A, B6, C, K manganese potassium

Helps to improve skin health & reduces symptoms of aging

Anti-aging

Qualities
Cold & Moist

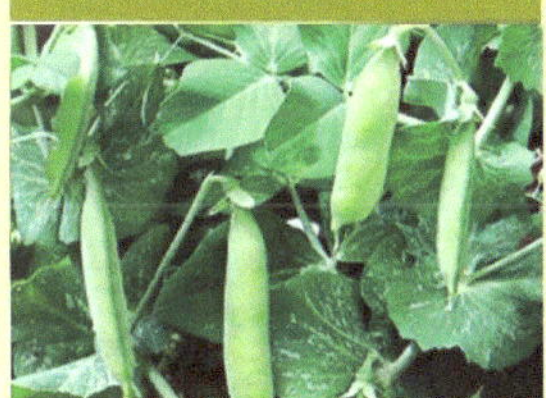

Prevents stomach cancer

Peas

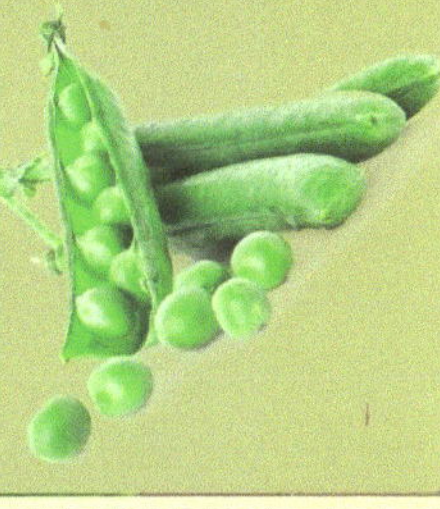

Immune booster

High in micronutrients

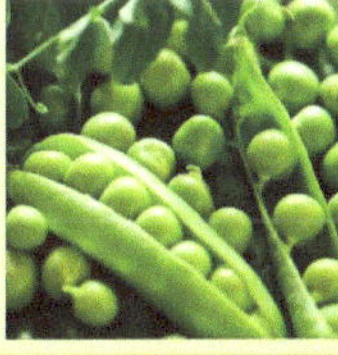

Regulates blood sugar

Aids liver function

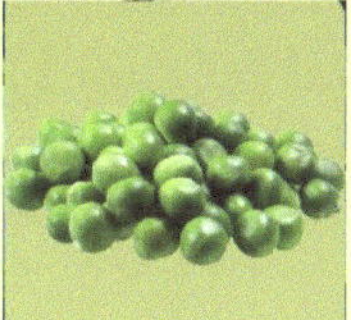

Guidelines for Eating

- Proper diet involves not just what you eat, but also when, how and how much

- Never eat when you're tired, angry, upset or worried.

- Fatigue, negative emotions and stress impair proper digestion.

- Don't eat unless you're truly hungry.

- Eat your largest meal at midday.

- Eat lightly for dinner, at least three hours before bedtime.

- A little light exercise before meals stimulates the appetite and digestion.

- Drink the most water between meals; sip while you sup.

- Don't overeat. Never fill your stomach past three- quarters full.

- Chew your food well before swallowing. Never eat on the run

- Eat in good company; make meals a happy, joyful occasion.

- Eat at least 5 servings of vegetables every day.

- Eat at least 2 servings of fruit every day.

- Drink plenty of water every day and limit drinks with added sugars.

- Don't shop when you're hungry – and use a list.

- Make meal times special occasions for the whole family.

- Don't spend a long time sitting down.

- Go for a walk, play active games, go for a ride, start a vegetable garden. Get the kids involved too.

- Buy fresh produce in season – for better value, availability and quality.

- Choose a variety of colors of fresh vegetables and fruits: green, orange, red, yellow, purple and white. Try new foods.

- Eat at home more often. Try new recipes and invite some friends, enjoy good food together!

- Eat whole-grain, high-fiber breads and cereals.

- Reduce daily intake of salt or sodium and sugar.

- If you drink alcoholic beverages, do so in moderation.

- Drink only when it doesn't put you or anyone else at risk. Learn to manage your stress with exercise, healthy eating, relaxation, and good coping skills.

Four Temperaments Test

Inventory (1) Moist qualities

Questions	Disagree	Occasionally	Agree
My skin is soft			
I like dry air and no humidity			
I am overweight			
I have soft and straight hair			
I sleep too much			
I experience memory loss and forget things			
I do not stay angry for long			
I am not rigid, I am flexible			

Inventory (2) Cold qualities

Questions	Disagree	Occasionally	Agree
I feel cold and my skin is cool			
I enjoy the warm and summer			
I have thin and light hair			
I have narrow shoulders and small chest			
I do things slowly and calmly			
I talk slowly and taciturn			
I do not get angry very quickly			
I am a cautious/timid person			

Inventory (3) Warm qualities

Questions	Disagree	Occasionally	Agree
My skin and body feel warm			
I enjoy the cool and winter			
I have black/dark hair			
I have wide shoulders and wide chest			
I do things with speed and acceleration			
I speak quickly and am talkative			
I get angry very quickly			
I am bold and brave person			

Inventory (4) Dry qualities

Questions	Disagree	Occasionally	Agree
My skin is dry			
I like humid air			
I am thin			
My hair is dry and not straight			
I do not oversleep			
I have a good memory and remember everything			
I cannot relax when I am angry			
I am not flexible, I am rigid			

SANGUINES	CHOLERIC	PHLEGMATIC	MELANCHOLIC
Talkative	Outspoken	Deep feeling	Very quiet
Emotional	Optimistic	Moody	Calm and cool
Funny	Determined	Calm, cool,	Deep and thoughtful
Has energy	Hot-tempered	Lazy Critical	Shy
popular	Quick thinker	Insecure	Selfish
Forgetful	Intelligent	Sensitive	Hesitant
Very positive	Bossy	Indecisive	Serious
Easily	Productive	Idealistic	Stingy
angered	Goal-oriented	Hard to please	Accurate
Egotistical	Competitive	Introvert	Unenthusiastic
Interrupts others	Decisive	Self-centered	Negative
Compassionate	Headstrong	Pessimistic	Perfectionist
Lives in present	Frank	Depressed easily	Conscientious
Impulsive	Self-confident	Easily offended	Regular daily
Enjoyable	Independent	Loner	habits Aimless
Curious	Quick tempered	Self-sufficient	Spectator of life
concentrating	Workaholic	Self-sacrificing	Works well under pressure
Impractical	Self-sufficient	Introvert	Not aggressive
likes to play	Practical	Analytical	Stubborn
Easily discouraged	Activist	Lives balanced life	Worrier
Undisciplined	Outgoing	Orderly	Indecisive
Extrovert	Domineering	Hard to get	Sensitive to others
Refreshing	Strong-willed	excited	Artistic and musical
Spirited	Daring	Creative	Philosophical and poetic
Sincere at heart	Dislikes emotions	Good mediators	Adaptable
Weak-willed	Persevering	Detailed	Slow and lazy
Spontaneous	Bold	Discourages	Submissive to others
Delightful/cheerful	Persuasive	others	Easy going
Difficulty with	Too busy for family	Patient	Reserved
appointments	Daring, risk taker	Gifted (musically	Content
Difficulty keeping	Resourceful	or	Satisfied
resolutions	Insensitive	athletically	Pleasant
Wide-eyed and	Unsympathetic	Considerate	Teases others
innocent	Likes pressure	Watcher, not doer	Consistent
Sociable	Leadership ability	Likes behind the	Efficient
"Bouncy"	Sarcastic	scenes	Patient
Restless	Adventurous	Good leaders	Dependable
Disorganized	Holds a grudge	Suspicious	Listener
Good on stage	Aggressive	Respectful	Witty/dry humor
Changeable	Easily bored	Unenthusiastic	Faithful and devoted
disposition	Inflexible	Faithful friend	Low self-image
Loves People	Excels in	Brings peace	Too introspective
Has loud voice	emergencies	Introspective	Insecure socially
and laughs	Passion to win	Planner	
Disorganized	Great	Perfectionist	
	ambition	Scheduled	
		Unforgiving/	
		resents	

HERBAL TEA

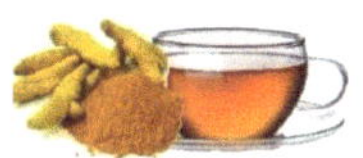

Turmeric

Regulate blood sugar
Lower inflammation
Ease arthritis
Lose weight
Protect against Alzheimer

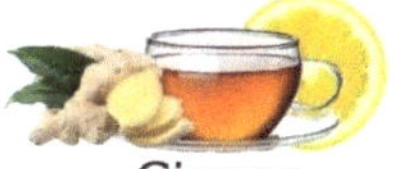

Ginger

Migraine Relief
Cold & Flu prevention
Reduces pain
colon cancer prevention
Reduces inflammation

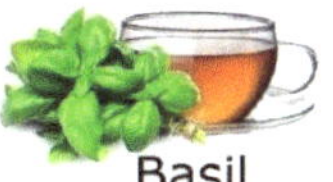

Basil

Eliminates Kidney stones
Prevents Acne
Cures stomach problems
Improves vision
Strss Buster

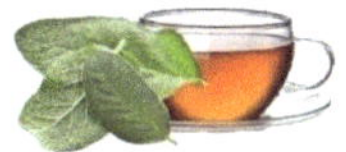

Sage

Eliminates scars
Digestive Aid
Cold remedy
Anti inflammatory
Diarrhea relief

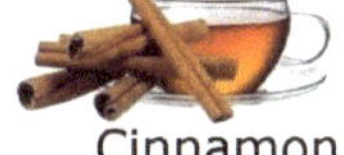

Cinnamon

Reduce blood pressure
Lowers cholesterol
Improves digestion
Blood sugar levels

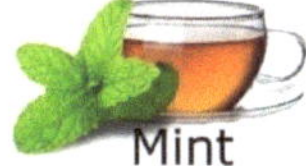

Mint

Promotes digestion
Help weight
Improves memory
Skin health
Relief coughs

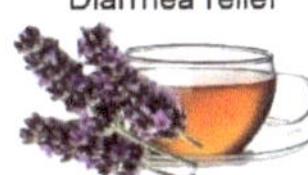

Lavender

Improves digestion
Relieves headaches
Helps asthmatics
Heals wounds

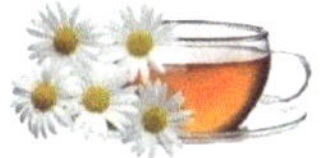

Chamomile

Digestive Aid
Menstrual pain
Cold relief
Help with diabetes

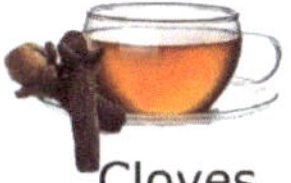

Cloves

Control high cholesterol
Helps gastric upsets
Avoids bloating
Fights tooth pain

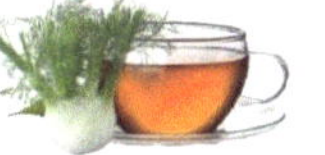

Fennel

Anti aging effects
Reduces obesity
Cardiovascular health
Nourishes the eyes
Soothes digestive tract

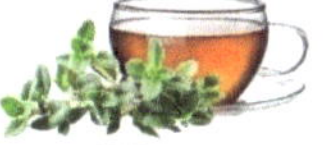

Thyme

Improves digestion
Reduce weight
removes toxins
Cure rheumatism
Cure arthritis

Hibiscus

Cure stomach disorders
Relief asthma
Aids indigestion
Remedy nausea & vomiting